SUCCESSFUL *NO CARBS AFTER 5PM* DIETERS

KATIE, 36: mum of 18-month-old Josh. 'The baby belly won't shift!'
Dropped 10 pounds and 6 inches off her waist.

TIM, THE DOCTOR, 42: 'But I've never had to diet before.'
Dropped 7 pounds and 5 inches off his waist.

STEPH, 34: mum of three children under five. 'I don't have time to exercise.'
Dropped 7 pounds and 5 inches off her waist.

BRONWYN, 28: newly married doctor and dedicated carb lover.
Dropped 5 pounds and 6 inches off her waist.

ZITA, 39: music manager and rock chick mum of four. 'I don't do exercise.'
Dropped 10 pounds and 7 inches off her waist.

HENRY, 58: retired property lawyer. 'You're never too old to party!'
Dropped 9 pounds and 6 inches off his waist.

CARMEN, 24: secretary, loves her social life.
Dropped 5 pounds, 4 inches off her waist and 6½ inches off her thighs.

JO JO, 36: businesswoman and mum of two, a diet cynic.
Dropped 7 pounds and 4½ inches off her waist.

TASH, 26: administrator and Aussie traveller, loves her food 'too much to lose weight'.
Dropped 4 pounds and 4 inches off her waist.

JUDITH, 68: ex-smoker, granny of seven. 'Tried every diet there is.'
Lost 10 pounds and 7 inches off her waist.

The NO CARBS AFTER 5pm Diet

By the same author:

Carb Curfew
Drop a Size in 2 Weeks Flat!
Drop a Size for Life
Drop a Size Carb and Calorie Counter

Joanna Hall

The NO CARBS AFTER 5pm Diet

with the NEW step counter plan

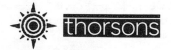

Thorsons
A division of HarperCollins*Publishers*
77–85 Fulham Palace Road
Hammersmith
London W6 8JB

The website address is: www.thorsonselement.com

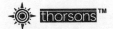

and *Thorsons* are trademarks of
HarperCollins*Publishers*

Published by Thorsons 2005

10 9 8 7 6 5 4 3 2 1

© Joanna Hall 2005

Joanna Hall asserts the moral right to be
identified as the author of this work

Joanna Hall's website address is: www.joannahall.com

Photography by Dan Welldon

A catalogue record for this book is
available from the British Library

ISBN 0 00 717529 9

Printed and bound in Great Britain by
Clays Ltd, St Ives plc

Contents

Introduction

Twenty-eight days is exactly four weeks. Just imagine: in four weeks you could have lost inches off your midriff. It is not impossible and you can do it. Twenty-eight days is just long enough for you to get great results. In less than a month you can change your body, lose inches off your waist, feel your fitness levels soar and fit into clothes that look great. Your health will improve and you'll enjoy so much more energy. In just 28 days...

I'm sure you've heard the Beatles' song *I Want to Hold Your Hand*. Life is full of hurdles and sometimes we need someone to hold our hand to give us extra strength. Losing weight and keeping it off is a hurdle. In this book I want to hold *your* hand as you follow my diet and exercise plan, giving you my advice and guidance every step of the way.

My *No Carbs After 5pm Diet* works! It is based on my 28-day Carb Curfew Plan, which I run in London. You can feel confident that you are following a programme that works and delivers results. It's been tried and tested in GP practices on men and women just like you. It has worked for them and I know it can work for you too. All you need to do is have some faith in me and in what I'm asking you to do, and give me a bit of commitment over the next 28 days.

The plan gives you clear information about what to do and why you are doing it. You'll find lots of tips from my successful clients along the way, as well as my advice and experience from running weight-management programmes. Your success will involve a little planning ahead, being prepared and becoming empowered. So if you want to follow a plan that works, drop inches off your tummy, lose pounds on the scales and feel fantastic in just 28 days – come on – let's get going!

Be active!

Joanna

1

How the Diet Works

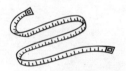

1

Setting the Scene

I am not going to wave a magic wand so you can experience the benefits of my 28-day diet without the effort. Putting in a little effort is very important for three reasons:

1 Making an effort means you value yourself. Achieving something with little or no effort often has no value and we don't really appreciate it.

2 The diet is simple to follow. You'll feel the benefits almost as soon as you start. What you may perceive as a little effort at the start of the plan will become part of a healthier lifestyle habit by the time you reach the finish line, without you even realizing it.

3 Your efforts will reap you major health improvements over the 28 days. As well as losing significant inches

and weight, participants have recorded decreased blood pressure, improved cholesterol levels, improved moods, better sleeping patterns, better sex and greater energy.

❝ You'll notice the difference in a week. The programme is *so* worth pursuing. My advice would be to get the first seven days done, and after that you'll find it quite easy to follow. ❞

At the start of every weight-management programme I run, the participants are always impatient to see their body change – they have heard about the fantastic results people have experienced and want to see and feel the benefits straight away. But we need to get one thing straight – and this is where the straight talking begins.

We may all have the *desire* to lose weight, to have that fabulous feeling of inches falling off, but the crux of the matter is how *willing* you are to fulfil that desire. Having the desire to lose weight and follow the programme will not get you anywhere without the willingness to put in a bit of effort. This means you will need to plan ahead a little, but I have taken all the hard work out and tried to make it easy for you.

WHAT WILL THE DIET DO FOR ME?

Many men and women have had fantastic success with the diet and I know you can too!

- ✪ **You will lose weight.**
- ✪ **You will lose inches.**
- ✪ **You will feel more energetic.**
- ✪ **You may benefit from lowering elevated cholesterol levels.**
- ✪ **You will be fitter.**
- ✪ **You will feel back in control.**
- ✪ **You may enjoy better sleep.**
- ✪ **Many people have reported having better sex!**

Everyone who has completed this programme with me has lost inches and felt fantastic.

" Lots of people have noticed the change in my body shape – I feel so much more sexy! "

HOW THE DIET WORKS

This diet is about getting results and making it work for you and the life you lead. It is a focused eating and walking plan designed to help you lose weight and inches, especially around your middle and waistline.

I am also concerned about you keeping the weight off long term. The National Registry of Weight Loss in Denver has compiled the details of people who have lost over 60 pounds in weight and kept it off for five years. And what is it that has helped these people succeed?

- They eat fewer than 2,000 calories a day.
- They average an hour of moderate-intensity physical activity each day.
- They don't follow fad diets or high-protein diets.

The principles of the diet and exercise plan are simple to put into practice. You'll soon see how they work and how easily they can be slotted into your life. The menu plans in Chapter 5 put all the diet principles into practice for you, but are flexible enough to adapt to your own preferences.

" I loved the flexibility and the fact that the plan is not a rigid regime where you have to eat this food at 11am and that food at 4pm. "

The exercise plan is based on walking and five tummy exercises. That's all – you don't need a gym membership, expensive exercise kit or flashy trainers, just a pair of comfortable walking shoes and enough space on the floor to do your exercises. And absolutely anyone can do it – I promise you.

The diet runs over 28 days. You can follow the 28-day plan strictly or take a more relaxed weekly approach, depending on what suits you. Throughout the book there are tips from me and many people who have followed the diet successfully, so you need not feel you are alone. The question and answer section in Chapter 15 addresses frequently asked queries. You'll also find lots of advice in the question and answer section of my website, www.joannahall.com

" The most important thing for me has been the fact that it isn't really a diet but more of a lifestyle change. "

Building a Template of Success

Being successful does require a little prior preparation. In the following chapters I'll outline how the plan works and how you can prepare for it. The easy-to-follow five-day countdown in Chapter 7 not only helps you get organized before you commence your 28 days to success but also gets you into the right mindset. This is vitally important and, in my experience, can be a deciding factor to you achieving your goals.

You deserve the best opportunity to have a fitter, healthier and slimmer body, but many individuals don't give themselves the right starting platform for success. They doubt their ability, feel guilty for taking the time out to feel better about themselves, or base their programme on previous diets that have been too rigid and impossible to fit in with their life. My whole programme is geared towards helping you achieve success whatever may be occurring in your life. Navigating the challenges life throws our way are all part of the programme. How you handle these and still achieve success is part of you feeling confident about the diet and about yourself. I call this building a Template of Success.

These little challenges can so often throw us off course, despite our good intentions. We can give up, thinking the time is not quite right, promising to start again soon. But the right time never seems to come, leading to feelings of frustration and building a Template of Failure, feeling you will never succeed. If this sounds like you, don't panic. 'Stop a Lapse Becoming a Collapse' on page 25 will keep you on track. You may also want to look at my book *Drop a Size for Life*, as this contains my seven-step approach to getting you in the right 'head space'.

DOING IT TOGETHER

I have written this book exactly as I run the programme, with tips and advice from me and my clients along the way. This should help you stay the course and feel the benefits my clients have experienced, and also make you feel you are not doing the diet alone. However, doing the diet with a friend or partner can be a real bonus, helping you get over the little hurdles and keeping you on track.

You can set up a little system with your buddy – why not text or e-mail each other your daily step totals, or set up a standard text message such as 'Carb Curfew successfully completed' when you have had your supper.

Choosing the Right Diet Buddy

Before starting the diet, people tend to anticipate that they will find it easier to implement either the exercise or eating principles. Once they get into the diet, however, they soon see how clear and simple both principles are to put into practice. You may find it best to buddy-up with someone who feels they will find it easier to implement the principles you expect to find harder. This matching will give both of you a boost when your motivation drops.

66 At first, John was quite obstructive and ordered Indian takeaways. But after a year of seeing me stick to the suppers in the evenings and thinking before I ordered in restaurants, he has now embraced the diet. Also, as much as people were telling me I looked good and had lost weight, they were telling him he had put it on! So by following Joanna's Carb Curfew he has since lost about two stone. 99

Keep it in the Family

Just about anyone can apply the exercise principles, so why not buddy-up with a family member. They don't have to live near you; arrange to e-mail or text each other your step tally. The pedometer is such a simple device that you can get the whole spectrum of the family involved: your children, parents, aunts and uncles. And because the targets are designed first and foremost to improve your health, everyone wins!

You and Your Loved One

When my female clients start doing Carb Curfew meals, many of them cook a few potatoes or some pasta or rice for their partner, thinking they will want it. What is interesting, though, is that the men soon see and feel the benefits of Carb Curfew, and naturally start to apply it themselves.

66 I did the plan with my friend and found having a bit of competition between us helped spur us both on. It worked well. We'd compare steps we did each day, and what lunch we had eaten. It gave me motivation when I needed it. 99

Coping with Kids

If you and your partner are doing the diet together, and you have children, you may find it harder to get the walking done in the evenings, especially if the children are too young to be left on their own. In this instance it may be more practical to have a buddy for your eating principles (such as your partner/husband) and another buddy for your exercise principles. And remember to get your children involved – let them be your walking buddies at the weekends, and allow them to fill in your charts and step targets. This can be a real motivator, and you are giving them a fantastic health message about looking after their own bodies too.

So if you are ready let's…

- ✪ **Plan ahead**
- ✪ **Be prepared**
- ✪ **Become empowered**

CLIENT FEEDBACK: ZITA

I have worked in the music industry for 17 years, running my own company managing producers, songwriters and artists. My job is very full-on. I have three children aged ten, eight and five. I also had a child adopted, who would now be 20. So, having had lots of babies, my stomach and navel area has always been the most problematic. After the first baby the weight just disappeared within weeks, but I piled on weight after each of the others. I gained four stone and looked like a womble!

When I went to have my annual medical recently, I found I had put on a stone without realizing it. My body fat was too high at 34 per cent, and my cholesterol was high as well. My doctor recommended Joanna's programme. He had followed it himself, lost over a stone and felt so much better. I have bad habits and drive everywhere. I've gone through phases of personal training but have never managed to exercise on my own before – until now.

I found the first week really hard. But once the endorphins start to kick in because of the walking and tummy exercises, I think that starts to make it easier. I just knew I was not going to stop after the first week.

I am a huge fan of Joanna's 28-day plan. I can't call it a diet – it really is a lifestyle change. I think that makes it easier in a way, as there's no beginning and end, just an ongoing programme. The Carb Curfew has kept my weight and inch loss constant. When I first started the programme, I really craved carbs in the evening. Now if I do eat carbs in the evenings, at other people's houses or at restaurants, I feel full very quickly, and often a little uncomfortable. I used to feel very heavy and tired after eating. I now feel light and have more energy. I love salads and have always enjoyed meat or fish and vegetables. The best thing is that if I stick to this I can still have my naughty treats during the day like crisps, a few squares of chocolate and an occasional slice of cake.

The exercising and the clear, easy-to-follow plan definitely affected my inch loss. I lost 6kg and 5 per cent body fat. My cholesterol went down from 6.75 to 5.5 in nine weeks, which was great.

Even with my busy lifestyle as a mum of three, running my own company, going out a lot and entertaining a fair bit, I have still managed to keep most of the weight off.

2

Recording Your Progress

CALCULATING YOUR BODY MASS INDEX

Recording your measurements is an important part of tracking your progress. Calculating your body mass index (BMI) will enable you to determine how much weight you need to lose. To calculate your BMI, divide your weight in kilograms by your height in metres squared. You'll find an automatic BMI calculator on my website, www.joannahall.com

⊙ **If your BMI is between 25 and 29, you are overweight.**
⊙ **If your BMI is between 30 and 39, you are obese.**
⊙ **If your BMI is 40 or above, you are morbidly obese.**

WHAT YOUR WAIST MEASUREMENT REVEALS

While BMI is widely recognized as a measure of obesity, it does not give a strong indication of your health risks. Storing your weight around your waist or midriff is known as 'abdominal obesity'. This measurement is much more closely related to your risks of developing chronic disease than your BMI value alone. So, on this diet, the number you need to know and are specifically going to track is your waist circumference.

Metabolic Syndrome

Metabolic syndrome is the term for a cluster of disorders that place you at increased risk of chronic disease. Your waist measurement is one of the strongest indicators of whether you are prone to metabolic syndrome and its associated disorders. These disorders include:

- ✪ **Excess levels of triglycerides ('bad' blood fats)**
- ✪ **Decreased values of high-density lipoproteins ('good' blood fats)**

○ **High blood pressure**
○ **A high fasting blood glucose value**
○ **Increased insulin resistance**

Waist measurements indicating risk of disease are different for men and women:

○ **Men with a waist measurement greater than 102cm (40 inches) are at risk.**
○ **Women with a waist measurement greater than 88cm (35 inches) are at risk.**

Please note: if a person has a short stature (under 5 feet in height) and a BMI of 35 or above, waist circumference standards may not apply. If this applies to you, ask your GP to assess your risk of metabolic syndrome.

Quite simply, the medical conditions that worsen with weight gain will improve with weight loss:

○ **High blood pressure**
○ **Dyslipidaemia (adverse blood fats)**
○ **Sleep apnoea**
○ **Infertility**
○ **Cardiovascular disease**
○ **Type 2 diabetes**
○ **Osteoarthritis**

TEST YOUR MOTIVATION

66 The motivation kicks in as soon as you start to see the results and realize you can maintain them. I felt results within four days. Also, quite early on, my skin felt better and people were saying I looked so much healthier. 99

Improving how we look is a strong motivator for us to take action and lose weight, but our health is important too. To test your motivation to follow my programme, complete the table below.

Read through these medical conditions. If you suffer from any of them, tick whether you want them to improve or worsen. If you don't have these conditions, tick whether you would like to increase or decrease your risk of developing them.

I appreciate that no one wants their health to get worse. Despite this, some people refuse to face up to the impact their lifestyle is having on their health. I have found this chart useful with clients, serving to give them a wake-up call.

HOW MOTIVATED ARE YOU TO CHANGE?

Tick this column if you are happy to take no action to prevent this condition or see it get worse.	Medical condition	Tick this column if you want to reduce your risk of this condition or see it improve.
	High blood pressure	
	Sleep apnoea	
	Infertility	
	Cardiovascular disease	
	Type 2 diabetes	
	Dyslipidaemia	
	Osteoarthritis	

Look at the side of the box you've ticked and then take action. If you've ticked any of the columns on the left, give this book to someone else because this diet is about you getting healthier, losing weight and feeling better about yourself. If you want to do something about this then read on. We've got some work to do, but I'm here to help – so let's get going!

BODY MEASUREMENTS

Before you start my 28-day programme you will need to take the following measurements:

⊗ **Your weight**
⊗ **Your waist measurement**
⊗ **Your navel measurement (around the midriff level with your belly button)**

Record these measurements on days 1, 7, 14, 21 and 28 of the plan in the chart overleaf.

	WEIGHT	WAIST	NAVEL
Day 1			
Day 7			
Day 14			
Day 21			
Day 28			

You may also want to take additional body measurements, such as your chest, hips and thighs, so you can track your progress. Many of my clients have found this very motivating, as you will see your body change shape elsewhere too! Use the chart below to record these additional measurements. I suggest you record them on days 1 and 28 only as it's likely that changes will be slower here, although your clothes will most definitely feel more comfortable as you progress on the diet.

	CHEST	HIPS	THIGHS
Day 1			
Day 28			

Over the 28 days I will ask you to record your weight and waist measurements on the chart every 7 days. If you have a tendency to weigh yourself every day I'd strongly urge you not to do this when following my plan. Daily weight changes tend not to reflect real changes in body shape and are more reflective of shifts in fluid retention.

RECORDING YOUR FITNESS

Just as you record how your body measurements change, I'd also like you to record how your fitness improves. This can be done very simply, by walking a set distance as fast as you can and recording the time it takes you and your heart rate. You will need to do this test at the very start of the plan and also on day 28. You will surprised at how much your body can improve in just 28 days.

On my 28-day programme we walk as fast as we can for one kilometre. If you are a complete novice to fast walking and exercise I suggest you complete a timed walk for half a kilometre. Your route should be as flat as possible. The route I use is beside a park. One length of the park is 250 metres, so we walk the length of the park four times to complete a kilometre as fast as we can.

Before you start your timed walk, record your heart rate for one minute. This can be taken at your wrist or your neck. See the box on page 24 for information on how to do this. Take your heart rate for one minute immediately after completing the walk, and then again after one minute of recovery. Record your heart rate results and the time it took you to walk on the chart below. Take a piece of paper and a pencil with you to jot down your results, and fill in the chart when you get back home.

	DATE	TIME TO COMPLETE 1KM	HR ON COMPLETION	HR AFTER 1 MINUTE
START Day 1				
END Day 28				

HOW TO TAKE YOUR HEART RATE

You can take your pulse either at your wrist (radial pulse) or at the side of your neck (carotid pulse). You can feel your radial pulse by tracing a line down from the base of the thumb. Place the tips of your index and middle fingers over the artery and apply light pressure.

Some people find it difficult to locate their radial pulse. Your exercise pulse, in particular, is much easier to locate at the carotid artery, to the side of the larynx. Do not apply heavy pressure to the carotid arteries because they contain baroreceptors that sense increases in pressure and can slow the heart rate.

Another very accurate and easy method of measuring your heart rate is with a portable heart monitor. There are a number of these on the market and they consist of a chest strap with electrodes that pick up the electrical activity of your heart. These are generally a lot more accurate as they are picking up your actual heart rate as opposed to your pulse.

THE DAY CHARTS

For every day of the 28-day plan, there is a chart to fill in. The day charts are easy to follow. They allow you to track the progress you make in both your eating and your exercise.

66 Writing everything down in the food diary may seem a hassle but it's the best way to ensure you are being totally honest with yourself. It may not be a coincidence that the first week, when I was most diligent in writing food down as I ate it, was the week I lost the most weight! 99

Recording What You Eat

All you need to do is record what you eat and tick the portion distortion symbols to keep your calories on track! It's that simple.

Here's what you do:

Each day record your breakfast, lunch, dinner and snack on the chart. You can select meals from the menu plans in Chapter 5 or fill in your own choices applying the eating principles in Chapter 3.

BREAKFAST AND LUNCH

Choose one from the breakfast and lunch suggestions. Each breakfast and lunch contains fewer than 400 calories. The breakfast choices are made of foods that release energy slowly so you will keep your hunger at bay right through to lunch. The lunches are made up of some protein, starchy carbs and at least two portions of fruit and veg.

DINNER

Choose one of the quick and easy-to-prepare 'Carb Curfew' meals on page 205 and serve with two portions of veg.

SNACKS

You can choose any snack you wish but it must contain no more than 150 calories. In addition, you need to drink a pint of skimmed or semi-skimmed milk. This provides you with an important source of calcium, which has a crucial role to play in helping your body fight fat. You'll find more about this in the eating principles on page 50. A pint of skimmed milk will provide you with 150 calories. Even if you don't like skimmed milk and can only drink semi-skimmed, it will still provide you with only 180 calories.

❝ The food diaries were especially useful to me. Filling them in gave me a real sense of achievement. ❞

WATER TALLY

Water is a vital component of our diet, and most of us don't drink enough of it. We often read that we should be drinking 2–2½ litres a day, which sounds a lot, but this can come from fruit, vegetables and soups as well as from water and other liquid foods. To put things in perspective, the British Olympic Committee encouraged athletes to drink 8 litres a day to avoid a decrease in performance during the Atlanta games.

However, like anything else, drinking more water than you need does not increase its health benefits. Indeed, drinking excess water can cause a dangerous condition called hyponatraemia.

To spread your water intake through the day, try to drink two glasses of water before or with each meal. Simply tick the box each time you have a glass. The water tally column will naturally guide you to consume eight glasses a day, but if you drink more simply add these to your drinks section of the chart.

PORTION DISTORTION

The portion distortion symbols are your easy calorie-control guide. Simply tick the symbol that represents the size of the food item you have eaten. If you eat more than one portion size of a food, you'll find space next to each symbol to record how many more servings you eat.

❝ Portion distortion has changed my life – I've never felt better. It's so clever, simple and easy to do that no one need ever know you are following a diet! ❞

When to Fill in Your Daily Chart

The most important aspect of filling in your charts is to be accurate. I know filling them in may seem a chore, but it really will make you focus on the plan.

In my experience with clients, the more time you leave between eating and recording, the more errors occur. So do try to keep this book with you so you can record at each meal. If you find this book a bit bulky to carry around, visit my website and print off these charts for free. Then you can keep them in your handbag, on your desk or on your PC!

Another approach I have found very effective with clients is to write down what you plan to eat for the whole day at the start of the day. This can be particularly helpful if you are the sort of person who tends to get very hungry before meals and grabs things on the run to stop the hunger pangs and energy slump. Filling in the chart this way will mean you need to be more organized but more focused. If you record what you plan to eat in one colour and then add any other food you have eaten in another colour, you can easily keep a hold on reality.

PREVIEW AND REVIEW CHARTS

On days 1, 7, 14, 21 and 28 you need to complete your preview and review charts.

Preview Charts

These help you plan your week ahead. They guide you to plan when you will be able to take your structured walks and do your abdominal exercises. They also address the difficulties you anticipate over the next seven days that may hinder your efforts.

Previewing is so important. I'm in no doubt you will come across a few challenges over the 28 days – maybe you are going to a huge blow-out party, it's your child's birthday tea party, you have deadlines at work, or an ill family member needs care. This is life, and how you deal with these events is part of your road to success.

The first thing to do is acknowledge them by writing them down in the Challenges section of your Preview chart, and perhaps to adjust your walking goals and times when you can commit to doing your abdominals. Remember, the 28-day plan is about building on a Template of Success. Over-committing yourself will only make you feel like you have failed.

Next, tick which of the following categories you think the following week will fall into: 'progressive', 'maintenance' or 'damage limitation'.

A **progressive** week is one where you feel 95 per cent confident you can complete all the aspects of the plan you have committed to on your Preview chart. You feel good about yourself; you feel motivated that you have planned ahead and happy that you can deal with any little blips that may come your way that week.

A **maintenance** week is one where you feel 75 per cent confident that you can complete your programme goals for the next seven days. You feel you may not be able to achieve all the daily walking goals, and you may have a few things to deal with that could make it difficult to follow the plan exactly, but you feel you can give it your best shot. You are confident that these little blips are not going to make your efforts lapse.

A **damage limitation** week is one where you feel your life is not conducive to following the plan – perhaps the children are breaking up from school, the washing machine has flooded the floor, it's your time of the month, you have major hassles at work and you have guests all weekend. Damage limitation weeks happen – you do need to acknowledge that – but rather than thinking 'I'll drop the plan this week, have a complete rest and pick it up again next week', DON'T! Limit the damage and pick one thing on the plan you can do all week. Perhaps it's your Carb Curfew or your daily accumulated walking targets, completing half the daily walking goals instead of all of them. Think carefully and plan – you can limit the damage, and this is all part of building that Template of Success The first step to limiting the damage is acknowledging it is a damage limitation week on your Preview chart.

66 I am not the most motivated of people so I found the weekly review and preview helped keep me on track. 99

Navigating all the challenges life throws your way is actually a success. OK, you may not always be able to complete the daily walking goals but the aim is for you to do something each day and feel good about it.

This is success and this is building on your Template of Success. Many of my clients have blips on the programme when they aren't able to do all the daily walking goals they wanted or perhaps slipped off the eating principles, but the trick is not to let a little *lapse* become a *collapse*. Even if you have a lapse, you will still see a huge difference in your body if you stick with the plan (see page 255).

Review Charts

These allow you to look back over the past seven days and see how you did. They encourage you to give yourself a pat on the back with your progress but, equally, to assess whether what you are expecting from yourself is realistic. Perhaps you ticked that you would do your abdominal exercises every day in the previous Preview chart on day 7. When you come to review it on day 14, however, you find you didn't actually do your abdominals *once*. This means you need to reassess how you fill in the Preview chart for the following week. The Review and Preview charts act as a reality check, keeping you on track and building a Template of Success. You'll find lots of ideas on how to deal with challenges and to stop a lapse becoming a collapse in Chapter 12.

THE ENERGY GAP

If you want to lose weight you have to create an 'energy gap' – put simply, you need to create as big a gap as possible between the number of calories you consume through food and drink and the number of calories you expend through moving your body. The amount of calories you consume through food and drink needs to decrease while the amount of calories you expend through moving your body has to increase. The bigger the energy gap you create on a consistent basis, the greater your success. *The No Carbs After 5pm Diet* will help you create an energy gap, with simple-to-implement exercise and eating principles. This will help you to lose weight and inches, and at the end of 28 days your body will burn more calories even when you are sleeping!

3

The Eating Principles

The No Carbs After 5pm Diet is based on a number of eating principles. Knowing the logic and science behind the diet will help you understand how and why it works. To make things simple, all the meal suggestions and recipes in the book put these principles into practice for you.

PRINCIPLE 1: CARB CURFEW

This is your Golden Rule.

Carb Curfew means no bread, pasta, rice, potatoes or cereal after 5pm for your evening meal. You can eat them for breakfast, lunch and snacks but you can't eat them after 5pm. You just say no at this time! But don't panic: you aren't going to feel hungry as there are still plenty of satisfying foods to eat. For your evening meal you can choose from a variety of nutritious foods including lean meat and fish, fruit, vegetables, pulses, dairy products and essential fats. You will find a whole host of delicious and easy Carb Curfew recipes in Chapter 9. Once you've got the hang of my Carb Curfew you'll soon see how easy it is to adapt some of your favourite meals.

66 I noticed almost immediately that cutting the carbs after 5pm meant I was not nearly so hungry, and my cravings disappeared. This gave me so much confidence. 99

Why Does Carb Curfew Work?

Carb Curfew is a tool. It's not about saying carbs are bad for you. Carb Curfew does three essential things that help you get the inches off and the weight down simply and easily:

1. It helps you get a better balance of nutrients.
2. It helps you cut your calories without having to try too hard!
3. It reduces uncomfortable tummy bloating.

The Food and Drug Administration in the US recently reported that people are consuming significantly more calories than they were 20 years ago, and that these extra calories are coming from carbohydrates. Any excess calories you consume will be converted and stored as body fat if they are not burnt off through increased physical activity. Simply cutting out the carbs after 5pm will automatically help you reduce your calorie intake without having to count calories continually, or deprive yourself of some of the important carbs you can enjoy at breakfast and lunch. In addition, consuming slightly more protein than usual will help you stay fuller for longer.

Putting Carb Curfew into practice will also help you get a better balance of nutrients. Not only will you get more essential vitamins and minerals from fruit and vegetables in your evening meal, helping you to hit the recommended five portions of fruit and veg a day, but the whole plan is designed to optimize your nutrition without you having to work too hard.

Reducing tummy bloating is one of the quickest benefits you will notice with my Carb Curfew. Eating carbs after 5pm can cause uncomfortable bloating for several reasons:

As your body digests carbohydrates they are broken down into glucose and either stored in the form of glycogen in the muscles or converted into fat and stored in the fat cells. Your body prefers to store these starchy carbs as glycogen but to do this it has to store three units of water with every one unit of glycogen. The net result is a bloated, puffy tummy and uncomfortable clothes.

Bloating can also occur when you have gone too long without eating. When you do give your body some food, your digestive system goes into shock, there is a surge of excess enzymes and the pH balance of your digestive system is distorted, creating abdominal discomfort.

Without stating the obvious, bloating can also occur simply because you have each too much too quickly. One reason individuals overeat is because they are too hungry, and when they start to eat their body does not have the ability to register when it is satisfied as opposed to over-full.

Following the Carb Curfew eating plan will take care of your bloating for you. It has been designed so you do not go too long without eating. Your energy levels stay elevated as your calorie intake is more evenly distributed, giving your body the energy it needs when it needs it. This means you will actually burn off more calories when you exercise. Many people have marvelled at the fact that they no longer crave biscuits and sugary processed snacks. If you follow the plan I am confident you will feel the benefits too.

PRINCIPLE 2: FRONT-LOAD YOUR DAY

Starving yourself all day in the perception that you are saving yourself calories is false economy. Eating too little by day only leads to overeating at dinner. Clinical studies may show that it makes no difference to weight loss if you eat your allocated daily calories in the morning or later in the evening. However, the participants in these studies have been in a confined environment with no fridge calling them and no free easy access to food in the kitchen!

In my experience of working with individuals keen to lose weight, starving yourself all day is a recipe to gain weight, not lose it. When you are hungry you will find yourself unable to make sensible food choices; you will find it difficult to identify when you are full and when you are stuffed, and the burden of excess calories on your digestive system is more likely to make you feel sluggish, lethargic, bloated and inactive. In addition, you will probably have to drag yourself through your daily walking tasks, and possibly even cop out – purely because you felt you didn't deserve to eat and were saving yourself some calories!

So front-loading your day not only makes you feel better and gives you more energy but also helps you burn more energy.

Front-loading your day is about getting food when your body needs it. My menu plans make this easy for you (see Chapter 5). The breakfasts and snacks are quick and easy to prepare, and you can choose from a whole selection of different lunches.

66 **Knowing that I'm not going to eat carbs for supper means I don't worry about having something at teatime such as a couple of biscuits and some fruit or a toasted teacake. This keeps me going until well into the evening because I'm not desperately hungry. 99**

Carb Curfew and front-loading your day work together so you wake up hungry, ready for your breakfast. If you have stuffed your face the night before, you will wake up with a 'food hangover'. The last thing you want is to enjoy your breakfast, so the whole cycle begins again, creating a bottom-heavy weight-gain day rather than a front-loaded weight-loss day.

A weight-gain day:

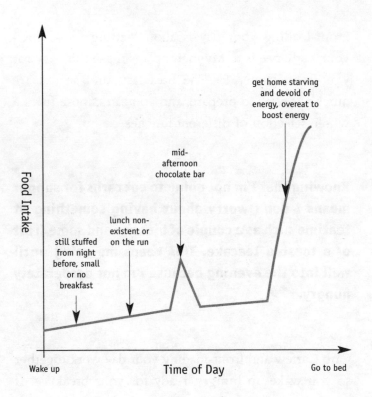

Net effect:

Total calories high. Calories highest when body calorie needs lowest.

A weight-managing day:

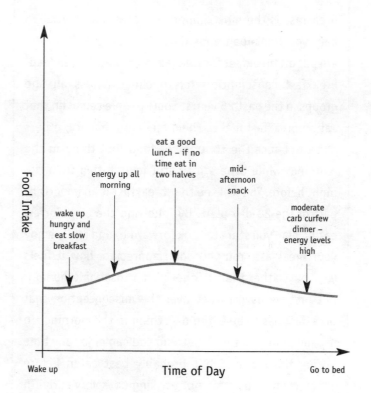

Net effect:

Total calories level but energy levels high all day – improving concentration and enabling you to do structured exercise.

THE IMPORTANCE OF BREAKFAST

Breakfast is the most important meal, and crucial to help you front-load your day. Many people, however, are put off breakfast for one reason or another. Indeed, breakfast consumption has declined across all age groups in the past 25 years. Some people complain that eating breakfast makes them feel more hungry; others just can't face the thought of food first thing in the morning; while others may still feel stuffed from the night before. You will see that breakfast is an important part of the 28-day plan. By following the Carb Curfew eating plan you start to look forward to and really enjoy your breakfast. You will soon appreciate how it fuels your day rather than triggering an insatiable hunger. But first we have to get over the misconception that breakfast has to be eaten first thing in the morning. To my mind breakfast is something you can enjoy any time during the morning but probably best eaten before 11am. Many of us start our working days very early. In this situation I suggest you either have two smaller breakfasts or save your breakfast and have it a little later in the morning.

PRINCIPLE 3: STOP PORTION DISTORTION

One of the main reasons we are gaining weight is simply that we are overeating. Trying to cut back can be a challenge as it is easy to misjudge the amount of food we actually eat. Also, in an attempt to cut calories we can get into the habit of omitting whole food groups that provide us with important nutrients.

Food manufacturers and fast-food outlets have been criticized recently for increasing the sizes of their portions. In the past 20 years, portion sizes have increased eightfold. Fierce competition between food manufacturers has led to portion sizes getting larger in an attempt to convey more value for the consumer. How much food you eat is an individual choice but when serving sizes are getting bigger and bigger it becomes increasingly difficult to decide what is a normal portion! 'Supersizing' is now considered to be the norm.

Trying to eat smaller portions can be difficult – weighing out 80g of meat or fish can be a bore – so let's make things simple! All you need to do to keep your meals in check is compile a handy 'portion distortion basket' in your kitchen. In the basket you'll put some everyday items that visually represent the correct portion size of a type of food. Seeing exactly what 80g of meat or fish looks like is so much simpler to put into practice than getting your scales out each time. You'll also find that this method works wherever you are – in a restaurant you can order what you want but eat only to the size of the portion shape on your plan. If self-control is going to be a problem then order a starter portion or share with a friend.

WHAT TO PUT IN YOUR PORTION DISTORTION BASKET

PORTION DISTORTION ITEM	USE FOR THESE FOODS	WHAT IT DOES TO YOUR BODY
Golf ball	Nuts and cheese	Provides a very dense source of energy
Deck of cards	Meat and fish	Builds muscle; important for burning calories and healing
One die	Oils and fats	Densest source of energy your body can consume
Tennis ball	Vegetables	Vitamins, minerals and antioxidants
Computer	Starchy carbs (pasta, rice, potatoes, cereal)	Fuels muscles for daily activity

66 Carb Curfew was so easy, and as long as I followed portion distortion I found I really could eat whatever I wanted. 99

The other great thing about portion distortion is that you can start the 28-day plan without thinking you have to deprive yourself of your favourite foods. If you want to have some chocolate you can, but eat only the specific portion size, which in this case is one die.

So grab yourself a basket, put all these items in it and keep it where you prepare your food. It's really important you do this: looking and cross-referencing the portion size helps keep you on track and acts as a prompt to remind you of your commitment to *The No Carbs After 5pm Diet*.

PRINCIPLE 4: GET YOUR CALCIUM

There is a growing body of evidence that calcium can play a crucial role in our attempts to achieve healthy weight loss. Although the specific scientific mechanisms are not as yet fully understood, it is thought that people with low calcium intakes have an increased ability to store excess calories as body fat. High levels of dietary calcium, on the other hand, can increase your body's ability to burn fat.

The calcium mechanism is thought to relate to the effect calcium has on insulin. High insulin levels tend to cause excess dumping of fatty acids in the fat cells. And if the diet is low in calcium it appears the fat cells send a signal to increase their production of fat. In addition, very high-protein diets may cause calcium losses from the body, which could adversely affect bone health and potentially damage the kidneys. It seems that maintaining a high level of dietary calcium is important for weight management.

How Much Calcium Should I Get?

Initial studies suggest a dietary intake of 1000mg of calcium a day. Indeed, in one study, men given 1000mg of calcium a day lost an average of 8kg. Another study showed that a high intake of calcium (1200–1300mg a day) was associated with significant inch loss from the abdomen and waist. The *No Carbs After 5pm Diet* gives you 1000mg of calcium each day in the form of a pint of skimmed or semi-skimmed milk. Drinking milk is also a great health message to give your children, as studies have shown that children who have a high intake of calcium and vegetable fat have lower body fat.

From a practical point of view, I have found drinking milk to be a very good weight-loss tip. I would specifically advise you to use it as part of your snacking. First, while it is a great source of calcium it is also a good source of protein. Protein sends a response to the brain triggering the release of dopamine, which makes us feel more alert. Second, drinking milk is very satisfying; the volume you consume will stretch your tummy muscles, making you feel full. Many of my clients have commented on how having a large glass of milk mid-morning and mid-afternoon has really helped stop their cravings.

GLASS TIP

Switch your short fat dumpy glass to a tall thin one – a recent study revealed that people who drank their fluids from a tall thin glass poured 40 per cent fewer calories than those who drank from a short fat glass!

What If I Don't Drink Milk?

The good news is that it doesn't matter what your sources of calcium are – so if you really hate milk, substitute it with unsweetened soya milk or take a calcium citrate supplement twice a day, morning and evening. While calcium citrate has the highest levels of absorption, taking more of it will not help your weight loss. In fact, taking too much (in excess of 2500mg a day) can actually soften your tissues.

A WORD ABOUT FIZZY DRINKS

Although the odd glass of pop can be really enjoyable, fizzy drinks can be high in sugar. They also contain phosphorus, which discourages your body from holding on to the calcium it needs. So try to avoid fizzy drinks as far as possible.

PRINCIPLE 4: ENJOY THE RIGHT CARBS

When it comes to giving you energy, carbs such as grains, fruits and vegetables are the hands-down winners. The popularity of low-carb diets has given carbs a bad name, but there is no refuting the available science. Your muscles are fuelled with glycogen, which is a form of the carbohydrate glucose – another name for sugar. In addition, your body needs carbs to burn fat as a source of energy when you exercise – so cutting out all carbs is not a good idea. Getting the right carbs is important for your energy and your health.

For many years carbohydrates have been divided into two types: 'simple' such as sugar and honey, and 'complex' such as bread and pasta. The message has always been that complex carbohydrates are 'good' and simple carbohydrates are 'bad'. However, the latest research suggests carbs are a bit more complicated than we thought. A system of classifying carbohydrates called the Glycaemic Index (GI) is turning some of the traditional ideas we have held about 'good' and 'bad' carbs upside down.

It has now been proven that if you eat a lot of foods with a high GI factor you have a greater risk of contracting both diabetes and heart disease. Consuming foods with a low GI value is thought to give you a slower release of glucose into your bloodstream, helping to keep your blood sugar levels more stable and minimize cravings. Some experts believe that eating low-GI foods may help the body burn fat more efficiently.

How Does the Glycaemic Index Work?

GI is a way of classifying carbohydrates according to the speed at which your body breaks them down and converts them to glucose to use as energy. The faster the food breaks down, the higher the GI factor (glucose has the highest GI factor of 100). Foods with a high GI are rapidly digested and absorbed and quickly raise blood sugar levels. Low-GI foods are broken down and digested more slowly, ensuring a slow and sustained release of glucose. Proteins and fats have little direct effect on blood sugars but, when eaten with high-GI foods, can actually slow down the glucose blood response, making a high-GI food behave more like a low-GI food.

If you eat a lot of high-GI foods your body is effectively overloaded with glucose. To combat this, the excess glucose which cannot be stored as glycogen is diverted to your bloodstream to be stored as fat. Remember: calories are calories whether they come from fat, protein or carbs!

GLYCAEMIC INDEX OF COMMON FOODS

LOW GI (50 OR UNDER)	MODERATE GI (50–70)	HIGH GI (70 AND OVER)
Yoghurt	Brown rice	White rice
Lentils	Bananas	Cornflakes
Apples	Sweetcorn	White bread
Kelloggs All-Bran	Couscous	Shredded wheat
Pumpernickel	Honey	Weetabix
bread	Sweet potatoes	Bagels
Porridge	Stoneground	Parsnips, carrots
Butter bean	wholewheat	Baked potatoes
Kidney beans	bread	Sports drinks
Chickpeas	Oatcakes	French fries
Milk	Raisins	Watermelon
Dried apricots		

Low-GI carbs are natural appetite suppressants; they are the best carbs to fill you up and control hunger pangs. High-GI carbs may give you an instant boost but often you will feel hungrier afterwards, which can mean you end up eating more! For staying power, combine your carbs with protein to keep your blood sugar on an even keel and to keep you moving. Your breakfast and lunches are based around low- to moderate-GI carbs. Don't feel you have to say 'no' to high-GI carbs for good, however. These are kept to a minimum on the diet, but where they are included I've combined them with a little protein and fat so they act like a low-GI carb as your body digests them.

PRINCIPLE 5: PICK THE RIGHT PROTEIN

Although many nutritionists are still wary about the potential dangers of high-protein diets, consuming slightly more protein than usual can be an effective tool for weight loss, as it helps you stay fuller for longer. *The No Carbs After 5pm Diet* is not a low-carb plan but based on a slightly higher intake of protein and a moderate intake of carbohydrate. All you need to do is make sure you eat some sort of protein at each meal.

Critics of high-protein, low-carb diets argue that they can result in a reduced intake of fruit and vegetables essential for vitamins and minerals, while the high intake of fat and saturated fatty acids could lead to a rise in blood cholesterol levels and an increased risk of heart disease. You'll see that my plan features a lot of fruit and vegetables and is naturally low in saturated fat.

While protein does not give you the same burst of energy you'll get from an orange or a slice of whole-wheat toast, it does give you staying power. This can make a big difference when you are exercising. Protein helps blunt the rise in blood sugar after a meal or snack, which aids in extending energy. Each meal in

my plan contains protein, with carbs and protein con-
sumed at breakfast and lunch and no carbs after 5pm.
Good sources of protein include low-fat dairy products, legumes, nuts and nut butters, lean red and white
meat and fish.

Eating protein after exercising can also help stimulate
muscle building. This has a direct effect on improving
your body's ability to burn fat.

Limit Fats

Eating excessive fats and a diet high in animal fats is not
only bad for your health but will also make you feel
more sluggish. Fats are the densest source of calories
your body can consume, with 1 gram of fat providing
9 calories. If you think of that in terms of a teaspoon,
1 teaspoon of olive oil gives you 45 calories!

Fat is the last nutrient to leave the stomach. It slows
down your digestion, leaving you feeling lethargic and
inactive. When you eat anything, the act of digestion
requires the body to increase circulation to the digestive tract. You really don't want your body to be digest-
ing food when your muscles are calling out for the

blood to deliver oxygen to produce energy for exercise and burn fat.

But don't cut out all fat. A little fat — especially omega-3 fats from fish oils and monounsaturated fats — blunts the rise in sugar. Essential fats are also helpful for your body in other ways. Research suggests that antioxidants in essential fats can help reduce the inflammation and stress that exercise puts on your body. To fully unlock their power, make sure you are eating enough good fats. Twice a week, aim to select a Carb Curfew dinner containing fish rich in omega-3s such as salmon, mackerel or trout. You'll find quite a selection of recipes in Chapter 9.

SUGAR ALCOHOLS

There is increasing evidence that sugar alcohols, also known as false sugars, are bad for your health and a long-term hindrance to weight loss. It is thought that they actually stimulate the body to store fat and can increase your appetite. You may have come across these false sugars in many diet foods. Feeling hungry and craving more sweet things is not going to help you on the plan, so try to avoid these sugar alcohols as much as possible.

All of the following terms found on ingredients labels are types of sugar:

Sucrose, maltose, lactose, dextrose, fructose, glucose, sorbitol, mannitol, glucose syrup, corn syrup, golden syrup, disaccharides, monosaccharides, polysaccharides, modified carbohydrate, raw sugar, brown sugar, molasses, honey, treacle.

CLIENT FEEDBACK: STEPHANIE

I've tried so many diets in the past, but what I really liked about this plan was that it's not just a diet, it's a complete approach. Carb Curfew was so easy. As long as I put the portion distortion in action, I found I really could eat whatever I wanted. I loved the flexibility, the fact that the plan is not a rigid regime where you have to eat this food at 11am and that food at 4pm. But I also got a lot of comfort from the fact that if I did have a blowout I could follow the eating principles strictly.

This plan is brilliant – I've lost 3kg and 7 inches off my body. Since the 28-day plan I've lapsed a little, but I've kept up the Carb Curfew and the inches have actually stayed off. The Carb Curfew is so easy to maintain: mentally you feel you are in control and physically you don't feel bloated.

This is the first plan where I've lost so much so quickly and kept it off. On other diets I have always found mealtimes an ordeal, worried about what I was going to be eating or having to prepare something different for the rest of the family. But portion distortion means you don't have to weigh anything. I found it so simple. I also found that my cravings disappeared almost immediately, which gave me lots of confidence. The food diaries were especially useful to me. Filling them in gave me a real sense of achievement.

Weekends in our household are big social events – we love having people over, and life revolves around food. But I found that as long as I kept Carb Curfew going, then I'd get back on track on Monday. I can maintain a quality of life while making a great investment in my health. Lots of people have noticed the change in my body shape – I feel so much more sexy!

4

The Exercise Principles

Exercise is an important part of *The No Carbs After 5pm Diet* and creating that energy gap (see Chapter 2). But before you start panicking about how hard you have to work, relax – the exercise on the plan is simple, based on walking and just five tummy exercises. So all you need is a pair of good comfortable walking shoes and enough space on the floor to do your tummy exercises. You get to choose which walking and tummy programme is right for you and that's it – simple!

Just as there are a number of principles behind the eating programme (see Chapter 3), so there are a few principles behind the exercise plan. Understanding these principles will help you see why I am asking you to do these routines. Have faith in the programme and it will give you great results.

PRINCIPLE 1: MOVE MORE, MORE OFTEN

66 I am always so busy and I feel like I'm running from one meeting to another or running after the kids, but I've realized it's all in the car! I'm now much more aware of the 'move more, more often' principle – it's stuck in my brain! 99

If you have read any of my other books you will be familiar with my concept of 'navigating the 24'. This is all about increasing your overall activity levels right through each day rather than trying to bust a gut every time you exercise. The idea is to move more and to move more often, whether at work or in your leisure time. All these extra times you are more physically active do add up.

Think of it this way – there are 24 hours in the day and 7 days in the week – that makes 168 hours in each week. Let's say we have the luxury of getting 10 hours' sleep each night. This leaves us 98 hours when we are awake and able to be physically active. Let's suppose we exercise three times a week for an hour each time, as this is the amount we are generally advised to take and the maximum most people feel they can squeeze into a busy life. This leaves us with 95 hours when we can physically move our bodies.

What I am asking you to do is get a bit more physically active right through your day. Have a look at the table below and you will see that moving more and more often can actually be the foundation of your physical fitness and weight loss.

Moving more and more often is much easier than having to drive to the gym, get changed, workout, shower and drive home. Becoming more physically active right through each day means you burn a few extra calories each time you move and keep your metabolism revved up right through the day. In reality, this means you burn an extra 2 calories a minute. This may not sound much but when you add it up over 24 hours, 356 days a year, you soon notch up over a million extra calories annually!

WHY GYM VISITS ARE NO SUBSTITUTE FOR AN ACTIVE LIFESTYLE

Less active person	kcals
Get someone else to iron while you sit down	34
Get someone else to vacuum while you sit down	11
Prepare pre-sliced vegetables	3
Microwave a ready meal	3
Drive children half-mile to school	11
Drive three miles to work	24
Use lift to travel up four floors	1
Chat with colleagues for 20mins at lunchtime	26
Shop by internet	17
Watch TV for two hours	175
Mow lawn with power mower for 10 mins	50
Read newspaper for half an hour	34
Basic Total	**389**
Compensatory gym workout (60 mins)	403
REVISED TOTAL	**792**

On a representative day, the less active person uses 30 per cent of the calories of the active person. If the less active person compensates by going to the gym he or she still only uses 60 per cent of the calories of the active person who does not use the gym.

Active person	kcals	Difference
Iron for 30 minutes	77	43
Vacuum for 10 minutes	40	29
Wash, slice & chop veg	28	25
Cook for 30 minutes	67	64
Walk children half-mile to school	56	45
Cycle three miles to work	135	111
Climb four flights of stairs	11	10
Walk and chat for 20 mins	78	52
Walk 1 mile to shop and back	311	294
Take a brisk one-hour walk	336	161
Mow lawn using hand mower	68	18
Play with children for $\frac{1}{2}$ hour	94	60
	1301	**912**
No gym workout	0	-403
TOTAL	**1301**	

Energy costs are for a 10st (63.5kg) person.
Source: British Heart Foundation health promotion unit, University of Oxford.

PRINCIPLE 2: TAKE STRUCTURED EXERCISE

This is when you stick on your walking shoes and complete your daily walking goals. Taking structured exercise works in conjunction with moving more, more often, so even though my plan encourages you to be much more physically active throughout your day, taking time out to exercise is still important for two reasons:

1   It is your opportunity to improve your fitness. Moving more, more often through the day will contribute to your overall calorie expenditure but exercise intensity is important to impact your fitness and maximize your calorie burn. Following my daily walking tips and weekly walking goals will automatically make you increase your walking intensity.

2   You'll have more energy, you'll sleep better and you'll feel great! You will soon feel these other benefits as you progress through the 28-day plan. Feeling better about yourself is an important aspect of the plan. Many of us feel low from time to time, and one in four of us suffers from depression at some point in our lives. Regular physical activity is one of the best depression

busters around. We live in such a fast-paced world now, and structured exercise gives you little moments of 'me' time. It's an investment for yourself that no one can afford not to make.

Every day you need to set aside some time to do your structured exercise walks. Walking is the simplest, easiest and cheapest exercise you can do. Whether you are already pounding that pavement regularly or you are more familiar socializing with the sofa, the 28-day walking plan is suited to all. And, what's more, it delivers results. It will get you out the door, moving your body and cranking up your calorie burn. Working alongside my Carb Curfew plan, it will help you melt away fat and inches.

66 **It's very easy to kid yourself that you are doing exercise. I used to do a lot of exercise but it was not necessarily the right exercise to lose inches. With Joanna's programme I achieved a body shape I'd never had. I look better now than I did on my wedding day! 99**

PRINCIPLE 3: COMMIT TO DOING YOUR TUMMY EXERCISES

The abdominal muscles are one of the few muscle groups that can be trained each day. The flat, firm and strong abdominals provide stability for the whole of your body so training them every day is beneficial to your posture and your body shape. Don't worry if you can't commit to doing them every day – as long as you do them at least three times a week you will see the inches come off. They are so quick to do – it takes just 7 minutes to whiz through them.

It doesn't matter when you do your tummy exercises, whether it's first thing in the morning or before you go to bed. These tummy exercises are simple to perform, don't put strain on your neck and give you a firmer, flatter, trimmer middle. They are unique as each exercise targets the whole abdominal area in one go, tightening your midriff. The end result is you get a tummy that looks like you are wearing a corset – though without the discomfort! As well as getting a better-looking tummy, these exercises also strengthen your spine and back muscles, helping to improve your posture and reduce back pain.

CHANGING THE WAY YOU MOVE

If you are reading this and thinking 'But I'm already very physically active', I need you to do an activity audit. I'm not calling you a liar but I am asking you to consider exactly what you mean by an active day.

We often perceive ourselves to be far more physically active than we are in reality. Studies have shown that people tend to overestimate the amount of exercise they take by an average of 51 per cent! So your day may be active and you may feel tired at the end of it, but are you actually *physically active* or are you more *mentally active*. Managing your home and just keeping your life on track gives your brain a great workout — but what about your body and your muscles?

Or perhaps you are *geographically active* because you need to be in a number of different locations all in one day — this side of town and the other, taking your children to school, getting to work. All this involves some sort of movement but this may be mechanical energy from a car, taxi, bus, train, tram, escalator, lift! Think about it...

Remember you can achieve your walking goals with your structured exercise sessions, and you can accumulate your daily pedometer step targets with your lifestyle and occupation exercise:

Structured exercise: This is when you stick on your walking shoes and complete your daily walking goals.

Lifestyle exercise: This is the amount of physical activity you take outside of your job. It includes how you get to and from work, the activities you do when you are not at work and all your weekend time. Surprisingly, most people are actually less active at weekends than in their working week.

Occupation exercise: This is the amount of physical activity you take with your daily job. This will vary considerably between different occupations. For example, if your job is desk-bound, requiring you to be sitting for most of the day, your occupation exercise level will be low. But don't be deceived: even if you are out and about for most of the day with your work or daily activities, your level of physical activity can still be quite low due to you being more geographically active than physically active.

" I found this plan so motivating – before I have always dragged myself to the gym and not really enjoyed it. Now I feel better about myself, more alert and not so tired. The pedometer makes you so much more aware of how much activity you are doing. I work in a busy GP's surgery and am always up and down the stairs, so I thought I was active. **"**

2

The Diet in Practice

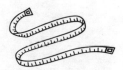

5

The Eating Principles in Practice

The No Carbs After 5pm Diet is easy. All you have to do is:

- ✪ **Select one breakfast, lunch and Carb Curfew meal each day from the lists in this chapter.**
- ✪ **Vary your meal choices to tempt your taste buds and provide your body with all the nutrients it needs.**
- ✪ **Snack on any fruit or sliced vegetables plus 570ml (1 pint) of skimmed or semi-skimmed milk.**

Remember: the recommended guidelines for fruit and vegetables are a minimum of five portions a day. Use your snacks to help you achieve this target. However, some people find eating too much fruit and veg makes them uncomfortable so aim for a maximum of five servings a day to avoid tummy discomfort.

❝ **The Carb Curfew is so easy to maintain. Mentally you feel you are in control and physically you don't feel bloated.** ❞

BREAKFASTS

All the breakfasts on the 28-day diet are carefully balanced, using low- or moderate-GI carbs, some protein and some essential fats. They are all designed to give you a slow release of energy right through the morning. Each breakfast contains fewer than 350 calories, but if you think having two smaller breakfasts will work for you, spilt the listed breakfast and eat half of it earlier and half a little later in the morning.

Choose one breakfast from the following list:

- ✪ 2 crumpets spread with 2 tsp almond butter; ½ pink grapefruit or glass of natural fruit juice.
- ✪ 2 slices wholemeal toast spread with peanut butter; glass of skimmed or semi-skimmed milk.
- ✪ 1 slice wholemeal toast spread with mashed ripe avocado; a boiled egg.

- Porridge (½ cup of oats with skimmed milk or water) topped with 1 tbsp wheat germ and handful of strawberries or raspberries.

- 2 slices raisin bread spread with low-fat cream cheese and natural, no-added-sugar fruit jam.

- Homemade Swiss muesli. Soak ½ cup porridge oats overnight with 1 grated apple, a small cup of soya or skimmed milk and pinch of nutmeg and/or cinnamon. Serve with small pot natural, low-fat bio yoghurt.

- Bowl of Special K cereal with skimmed or semi-skimmed milk; glass of orange juice or piece of fruit.

- Open bacon and tomato sarnie! Grill 2 slices of bacon and 2 tomatoes and layer on a slice of wholemeal toast.

- Small skinny latté coffee, skinny bran muffin and cube of reduced-fat cheese.

- Wholemeal toast topped with Marmite, sliced avocado and grilled bacon.

- 4 oatcakes topped with low-fat soft cheese or cottage cheese and salsa.

- Small bag of nuts and dried fruit, pot of natural bio yoghurt (preferably organic) and tablespoon of wheat germ – you can mix this all together if you need to eat on the run.

- Fruit salad; 2 Ryvita topped with 2 slices of cold ham and tablespoon of cottage cheese.

- ☼ Breakfast shake – blend 425ml (¾ pint) milk with ½ a small tin of pitted prunes, a handful of ice and a handful of bran flakes.
- ☼ Breakfast shake – blend 425ml (¾ pint) milk with any frozen fruit of your choice (e.g. strawberries, raspberries), 2 tbsp low-fat fruit yoghurt and a handful of ice.
- ☼ The chocolate one – dissolve 1½ small sachets of low-fat hot chocolate powder in a little hot water. Blend with 425ml (¾ pint) milk and a handful of ice. Piece of fruit.
- ☼ One small unpeeled banana frozen in chunks blended with 425ml (¾ pint) skimmed milk, a couple of ice cubes and 1 tbsp wheat germ.

LUNCH

The lunch options all contain some protein, starchy carbs, a little essential fat and some fruit or vegetables. Each lunch contains fewer than 400 calories. You'll find ideas that take under five minutes to prepare, as well as some that may be easier to enjoy at home. To make life even simpler I've included some of the Carb Curfew dinners. Make an extra portion the night before and simply add a starchy carb of your choice for a satisfying lunch.

Choose one lunch from the following list:

On-the-run Lunch Options:

These lunches take under five minutes to prepare so are great if you are in a rush or putting together a packed lunch.

- ✪ 4 low-salt crackers, celery, cucumber and carrot sticks and small pot (150g) of low-fat hummus.
- ✪ Full of Goodness (FOG) Soup (see page 252).
- ✪ Pitta bread stuffed with roasted vegetables and cottage cheese.
- ✪ Mixed Bean Salad with Parma Ham and Rocket (see page 214) salad served with small pieces of toasted wholemeal pitta bread.
- ✪ Summer Salad of Poached Salmon with Spinach and Mangetout and Minty Yoghurt Dressing (see page 224); small wholemeal bread roll.
- ✪ Golden Fish Chowder (see page 230) with small bread roll.
- ✪ Curried Mushrooms with Gingery Dhal and Creamy

Spinach (see page 239); wholegrain rice or wholemeal flatbread or pitta chips.

✪ Super-simple Vegetarian Chilli with Lime and Coriander (see page 250); ½ cup cooked wholegrain rice or small wholegrain bread roll.

Shop-bought Options:

Any shop-bought sushi under 400 calories plus piece of fruit.

Any shop-bought sandwich under 350 calories (no more than twice a week).

At Home Options:

✪ 2 poached eggs on 1 slice of wholemeal toast spread with Marmite.

✪ Bruschetta with rocket, Parma or good lean ham, 4 steamed asparagus spears and a side salad drizzled with a little lemon juice and olive oil.

✪ Open sandwich selection:
Take 1 slice of wholemeal bread, top with green salad and add:

- 2 slices lean ham, 2 tablespoons cottage cheese and peaches.
- Small tin of tuna – jazz it up with chopped tomatoes, fresh basil and drizzle of good olive oil.
- Mixed Bean Salad with Parma Ham and Rocket (see page 214).
- Couple of slices of cold roast chicken with half a sliced avocado.
- Rocket and sliced baby tomatoes topped with soft poached egg.
- Couple of slices of cold roast turkey plus cranberry sauce and drizzle of olive oil.
- Tinned salmon with sweetcorn mixed in 1 tbsp low-fat natural yoghurt and 1 tsp dried dill.
- Cooked prawns with natural yoghurt, fresh dill and cubed cucumber.

✪ Fresh vegetable soup; 2 Ryvita spread with ½ a mashed avocado and 1 tbsp cottage cheese.

✪ Scrambled eggs with smoked salmon on a slice of wholemeal toast; cucumber and dill salad.

✪ Seafood Stew with Tomato, Fennel and Orange (page 236) with small bread roll or ½ cup cooked wholegrain rice stirred into the soup.

✪ Chickpea Soup with Sun-dried Tomatoes (see page 248) with ½ cup cooked pasta shells, wholegrain rice or cooked barley.

CARB CURFEW DINNERS

Recipes for all the Carb Curfew dinners listed here can be found in Chapter 9.

Choose one Carb Curfew dinner from the list below or make your own supper using the Carb Curfew principles on page 38.

Meat

✪ **Sausages and Lentils with a Beetroot and Walnut Salad (see page 206).**

✪ **Pork Chops with Cannellini Beans in a Tomato and Mushroom Sauce (see page 212); steamed green beans.**

✪ **Mixed Bean Salad with Parma Ham and Rocket (see page 214).**

✪ **Griddled Chicken Breast with Roasted Vegetable Ratatouille (see page 220).**

✪ **Grilled Lamb Chops with Flageolet Beans and Rosemary-roasted Cherry Tomatoes (see page 209).**

✪ **Pork Chops with Baked Pears, Butternut Squash and Mint Vinaigrette (see page 216).**

✪ **Ham with Broad Beans in a Simple Parsley Sauce (see page 218).**

Fish

✪ **Summer Salad of Poached Salmon with Spinach and Mangetout and Minty Yoghurt Dressing (see page 224).**

✪ **Baked Fish with Steamed Leeks in a Crème Fraîche and Chive Sauce (see page 228).**

✪ **Golden Fish Chowder (see page 230).**

✪ **Grilled Mackerel with Apple Sauce and Spinach Salad (see page 232).**

✪ **Scrambled Eggs with Smoked Salmon and a Cucumber and Dill Salad (see page 234).**

✪ **Seafood Stew with Tomato, Fennel and Orange (see page 236).**

✪ **Baked Trout with Peas and Pesto (see page 226).**

Vegetarian

○ **Roast Butternut Squash with Smoked Tofu and Red Pepper Sauce; green beans (see page 242).**

○ **Speckled Salad with Lemon Feta Dressing (see page 246).**

○ **Chickpea Soup with Sun-dried Tomatoes (see page 248).**

○ **Super-simple Vegetarian Chilli with Lime and Coriander (see page 250).**

○ **Curried Mushrooms with Gingery Dhal and Creamy Spinach (see page 239).**

○ **Griddled Aubergine with a Green Salad and Lemon Feta Dressing (see page 244).**

CLIENT FEEDBACK: KATIE

I definitely used to have the same portions as my husband, but now I make a conscious effort to have less and fill the plate up with salad if I'm feeling deprived! Writing everything down in the food diary may seem a hassle but it's the best way to ensure you are being totally honest with yourself. It may not be a coincidence that the first week, when I was most diligent in writing food down as I ate it, was the week I lost the most weight!

I started the course because I had a 40th birthday party to go to at the end of the month and had bought a pair of trousers that were much too small – normally a big mistake. It certainly helped me to focus on the plan. I would try the trousers on every other day, and the fact that I could feel and see them getting looser was a great incentive. By the time of the party, not only did they fit but I needed the waist band taken in!

I am now the same weight (and probably a better shape) as when I got married six years ago.

6

The Exercise Principles in Practice

It's easy to put the exercise principles into practice. This chapter shows you how. All you have to do is:

- ✪ Use the following quiz to find out if you are a walking novice or walking whiz.
- ✪ Complete your daily walking goals in your structured exercise sessions.
- ✪ Increase your overall levels of physical activity.

ARE YOU A WALKING NOVICE OR A WALKING WHIZ?

You are a **walking novice** if:

- ✪ You take cardiovascular exercise *less than* three times a week for 40 minutes.
- ✪ Your job is relatively inactive, involving you sitting for most of the day.
- ✪ Your leisure pursuits are based around sedentary activities such as watching television.
- ✪ Your daily life is relatively inactive.

You are a **walking whiz** if:

- ✪ You take cardiovascular exercise *at least* three times a week for 40 minutes.
- ✪ Your job involves you being physically active, getting up and moving around at least once an hour.
- ✪ You have physically active hobbies, such as cycling or walking.
- ✪ You are constantly on your feet at home, doing jobs around the house.

Now that you have discovered whether you are following the Walking Whiz or Walking Novice programme, turn to Chapter 8 to find your personal walking plan.

WHY WALKING EXERCISE WORKS

Your motivation will fluctuate over the 28 days of the diet so understanding the logic behind what I am asking you to do is important to help you stay on track. Walking at a brisk pace will give you a calorie burn of approximately 5 calories a minute. Research has shown that achieving a calorie burn of 1,250 a week through physical activity will, in conjunction with the Carb Curfew plan, result in weight and inch loss. I've done all the planning for you – you can do this – so let's get a grip and go for it!

66 **I found it hard to embrace the diet during the first week, but once the endorphins started to kick in from the walking and tummy exercises, it started to get easier. I just knew I wasn't going to stop after the first week. 99**

USING A PEDOMETER

A pedometer is a great tool to accompany your walking plan, allowing you to record the number of steps you take a day. I'd strongly encourage you to invest in one. Your pedometer works by measuring the up-and-down motion of your hip as you walk. It will also measure movements you perform during your day in addition to walking, such as walking up and down stairs or getting in and out of your car. This is fine because activity can be accumulated from other forms of movement like these.

As long as you wear your pedometer correctly (see opposite), it will measure the actual number of steps you take to an accuracy of within 1 per cent. So if you take 100 steps, it should be no more than a step out. Different models have different levels of accuracy – the model which has been tested in independent trials to be the most accurate and easy to use is available from www.sportex.com

At the end of each day, take off your pedometer and write down the number of steps you've taken on your day chart.

How to Wear Your Pedometer

1 Slide the clip onto your belt or waistband. The most common position is directly above and in line with your knee. However, you may have to experiment to find the best placement for your body type. If your tummy protrudes over your waistband or belt, it may cause the pedometer to tilt and not work properly. If this is the case try wearing it more to the side of your body. Take care to position the pedometer in such a way that you are not likely to brush the reset button accidentally.

2 If your pedometer comes with a security strap, attach the strap's clip onto a belt loop, waistband or belt.

If you don't want to invest in a pedometer, you will need to aim to move your body for a set amount of time each day on top of your structured exercise walking tasks:

- ○ **30 minutes' moderate-paced walking = 4,000 steps**
- ○ **45 minutes' moderate-paced walking = 7,500 steps**
- ○ **60 minutes' brisk-paced walking = 10,000 steps**

WHAT IS THE SIGNIFICANCE OF 10,000 STEPS?

Evidence suggests that walking 10,000 steps a day can lead to significant health benefits. It can make you feel better and help reduce the risk of developing serious illnesses such as heart disease, some cancers, diabetes and depression. Put another way, the 10,000 steps message is merely encouraging you not to sit down for too long. If you get up and move every 30 minutes, you'll soon clock up those steps. In addition, getting into the habit of taking 10,000 steps becomes your foundation for your physical activity and exercise. When life gets busy, the first thing that tends to be put to one side is our structured exercise. When this happens, accumulating your 10,000 steps during your daily routine will still contribute to your overall calorie burn. Studies have shown that taking 10,000 steps a day will maintain your weight without the need to adjust your diet in any way.

❝ I love my pedometer. The daily walking targets kept me on track and became part of my everyday life in a very short time. ❞

WALKING TROUBLESHOOTING

Walking is the simplest form of exercise you can take – you just put one foot in front of the other! But there are a few tweaks to your walking technique that can help you get more out of your walking. A good walking technique will help you burn more calories, minimize your risk of any little aches and pains, and just make the whole experience a lot more enjoyable.

Technique Tips

WARM UP SLOWLY

Five minutes of easy walking can help you log more miles by warming up your muscles. Wrap up with five minutes of easy walking and you'll finish with a more enjoyable impression of your workout, making you less likely to skip it tomorrow.

KEEP YOUR HEAD UP

Keep your line of vision focused on what's ahead, and try not to look down at the ground. This decreases neck strain and improves posture.

In bright light or drizzling rain it is natural to tilt your head down to avoid the glare or the wet. To improve your walking posture, wear a hat or sunglasses so you can keep you chin up and parallel to the ground.

ROCK AND ROLL

For a more efficient, less jarring stride, visualize your feet as rockers on a rocking chair. Start each step on the heel and rock your foot forward until you roll onto your toes. Pick up your speed so you're rolling the foot with each stride.

Banish Aches and Pains

As you start your walking programme you may come across a few little niggles in your body. This is quite normal and to be expected if you are new to exercise.

However, to keep you walking stronger and longer and burning more energy, try these little tips to avoid common problems.

AVOID SHIN PAIN

Foot Roll

Standing with your feet almost together, roll up onto your toes, hold for two seconds and roll back down. Then roll onto the outside of your feet, hold both for two seconds and roll back down. Next roll onto your heels with the toes off the ground, hold for two seconds and roll back down. Do this sequence 10 times before every walk.

AVOID KNEE PAIN

Straight Leg Raise

Sit on the ground with your left leg extended in front of you, right leg bent and foot flat on the ground. Place your hands behind you and sit up straight. With your left foot flexed, contract your left thigh and raise your leg 6–12 inches off the floor. Hold for five seconds and then lower. Do 10 lifts, and then switch sides. Perform the sequence two to four times a week.

AVOID LEG ACHES

Hip and Calf Stretch

Standing with your feet together, step your right foot in front of you about 3–4 feet so both feet are pointing forward. Bend your right knee so it is just above but not in front of your right foot. Check both big toes are facing forward. Keep your left leg straight and your left heel on the ground to feel a stretch in your left calf. Flatten your lower back and tuck in your pelvis so you also feel a stretch in the front of your hip.

Hold for 4–7 slow, deep breaths, release and repeat on the other side. Stretch each leg two times after each walk.

Lower Calf Stretch

Stand close to a tree or lamppost and place the ball of the foot on the post or trunk so the heel is still on the ground but the ball of the foot is resting on the post. Bend the knee in towards the post; you should feel the stretch in the lower part of the calf. Hold for 10–15 seconds and repeat twice on each side. Do this at the end of each walk.

AVOID UPPER ARM TENSION

Upper Body Stretch

Stand with your feet about shoulder-distance apart. Raise your right arm over your head, bending your elbow so your right hand is behind your head. Place your left hand on your right elbow and gently pull your elbow to the left, allowing your upper body to bend slightly to the left.

Hold for 4–7 deep breaths, release and repeat on the other side. Stretch each side twice after every walk.

CHOOSING THE RIGHT TUMMY EXERCISES FOR YOU

Next, decide which level of tummy exercises is best for you. Choosing the right level is important; opting for harder ones than you are ready for can mean you don't perform the exercises correctly and don't get a flat tummy. Harder in this case does not necessarily mean you are going to get better results.

Choose the **No Neck Pain Programme** if you:

- ✪ **Are new to abdominal exercises**
- ✪ **Suffer from neck pain with your abdominal exercises**
- ✪ **Have a popped-out, domed belly, perhaps from performing abdominal exercises with poor technique**
- ✪ **Have just had a baby**

If you do a lot of abdominal work but feel frustrated with never getting the results you want, I'd suggest you follow the No Neck Pain Programme for the first week to help you really master the techniques, then move on to the advanced programme from day eight onwards.

Choose the **Advanced Abdominal Programme** if you:

✪ **Are familiar with abdominal exercises**
✪ **Have mastered the rib–hip connection**
  (see overleaf)
✪ **Suffer from no back or neck pain**

Once you have chosen which abdominal programme you are going to do, turn to either page 103 or page 110 to see your personal plan.

THE RIB–HIP CONNECTION

Once you have mastered this technique, you will start to see a real improvement in your abdominal training.

When you lie on the floor before starting abdominal exercises, make sure you have a connection between your ribs and your hips. This will help you contract the abdominals before you lift and ensure you are in the correct anatomical position for your spine. Here is what you do. Place your thumb on your bottom ribs and your fingers at the top of the hip bone. Draw these two points together with a small contraction of the abdominal muscles. Your spine should be in a neutral position. This neutral position will vary from person to person, depending on the shape of the spine. However, there should be a small space between the floor and your back. Keep the rib–hip connection so you maintain your neutral position to establish trunk stability.

Flat Abdominal Programme

NO NECK PAIN PROGRAMME

Exercise: Dead Bug

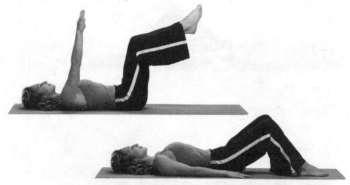

Lie on your back and lift your legs off the floor, so your knees are over your hips and your arms are directly over your shoulders. Hold this position for 20 seconds, keeping as still as possible and firmly pulling your abdominals into the base of your spine. Relax down for 10 seconds and repeat 5 times.

Joanna's Top Tip

Make sure your legs are not too close to your body, otherwise this becomes too easy. Experiment by extending the knees away a little so you feel some tension on your abdominals.

Exercise: Heel Slides

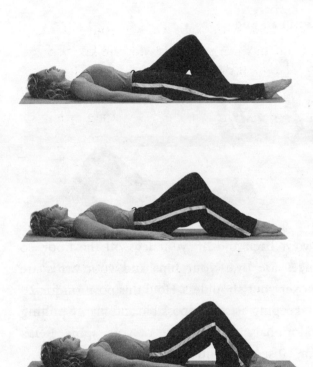

Lie on your back with your arms by your side, legs stretched out in front of you. Bend one knee so the foot is flat on the floor by the knee of the straight leg. Keeping your hips still, pull in your tummy muscles and slowly draw the heel of the straight leg in towards the other foot. Keep the foot relaxed and slowly extend the leg out along the floor again. Do this exercise 8 times for each leg.

Joanna's Top Tip

Keep the foot relaxed and focus on the tummy muscles, not the thigh muscles, drawing the leg in.

Exercise: Belt Pulls

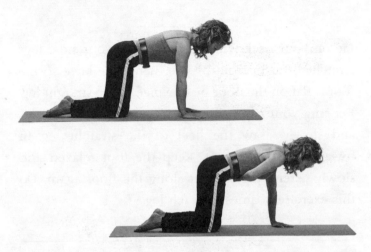

First put on a belt, buckling it so it fits snugly around your waist. Get onto all fours with your hands under your shoulders and your knees under your hips. Start with your abdominals relaxed; you may find your tummy is touching your belt. Now, keeping the back straight, draw in the abdominal muscles so you create space between your tummy and your belt. You should be able to slip your fingers between your belt and your tummy. Hold this position for 30 seconds, breathing smoothly throughout. Relax for 10 seconds and repeat 5 times.

Exercise: Belt Pull Balance

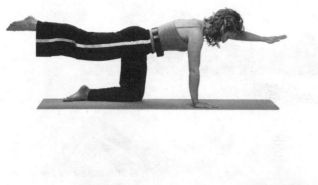

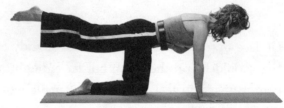

Start on all fours with your snug-fitting belt as above. Keep your back straight as you extend an opposite arm and leg. Now, draw in your abdominal muscles firmly to create the space between your belt and your tummy. This is more challenging than the previous exercise so start by holding this position for 10 seconds and build up to 5 sets of 30-second holds.

Exercise: Breast Bone Lift

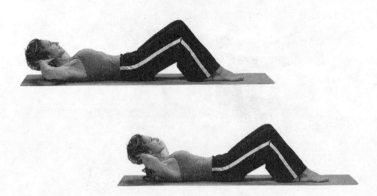

Lie face up on the floor with knees slightly bent. Your feet should be on the floor, but far enough from your bottom that you feel your toes are just about to come off the floor. Place your hands at the side of your head and lift your head off the floor. This is your start position. From here, lift no more than 10cm from the breastbone. Hold this small lift for 4 counts then return to the start position and lower the head to the floor.

Joanna's Top Tip

This is a very subtle exercise. Make sure you keep your abdominals contracted and pulled in throughout.

ADVANCED ABDOMINAL PROGRAMME

Exercise: Moving Dead Bug

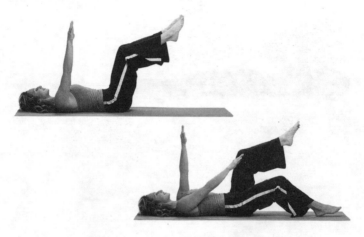

Start in the dead bug position: hands directly over shoulders and knees slightly extended to engage your abdominals. Slowly lower the same leg and arm towards the floor, keeping an equal distance between the hand and the knee. Gently 'kiss' the floor with your heel and slowly lift the arm and leg back up to the starting dead bug position. Repeat 12 times.

Joanna's Top Tip
Keeping the same distance between the arm and knee is crucial in this exercise. To help you, imagine you have a large beach ball between them.

Exercise: Full Roll Up

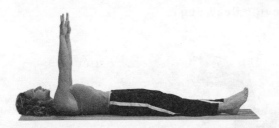

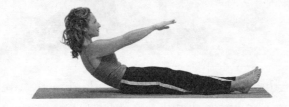

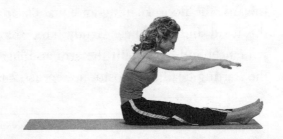

Start lying on the floor, legs extended straight out in front of you and arms directly over your shoulders. Slowly curl up one vertebra at a time, using your abdominals and not your legs. Keep the spine curved and your reach forward with your hands towards your feet. Sit straight with shoulders directly over hips and slowly curl down, one vertebra at a time. Repeat 6–8 times.

Joanna's Top Tip

This is a difficult exercise so you might find it easier to start sitting up and curl down first. Master this technique and then combine it with the rolling up and rolling down. Bending the knees a little also makes this exercise easier. Your thigh muscles will really want to help you sit up; to avoid this place a small cushion between your feet and squeeze it together hard.

Exercise: Ab Reach

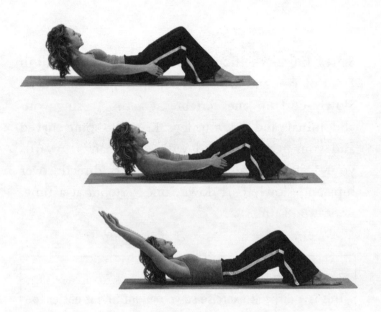

Start on your back with your knees slightly bent so that your feet are almost off the floor. Lift your head off the floor, leading from your breastbone, and place your hands by your thighs. This is your start position. Lift your head a further 10cm from the breastbone, trying to reach further around your thighs with your hands if you can. Lower back to your start position and extend your arms above your head, keeping your shoulders off the floor.

Exercise: Towel Oblique Reach

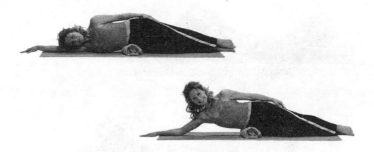

Take a large towel and roll it into a sausage shape. Lie on your side so your hip is placed on top of the towel. Make sure your hips are stacked up on top of each other, pulling in your abdominals tightly to avoid you toppling either forwards or backwards. You may need to play around with the towel position so you can use your waist muscles more as you lift. Extend your bottom arm along the floor and your top arm by your side. Keeping the waist long, extend out through the top of the head as you lift your body. You should feel your waist muscles tightening. Lower yourself slowly and repeat 8 times on each side.

Joanna's Top Tip

The arm on the floor is for support and balance. Try to avoid using it to push you up.

Exercise: Straight Leg Lift

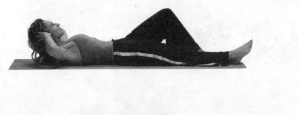

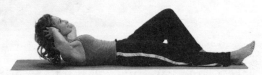

This is a variation on the breastbone lift but more challenging, with only one leg extended. Start with one leg extended. Place your hands at the side of your head and lift the head off the floor. This is your start position. From here lift no more than 10cm from the breastbone. Hold this small lift for 4 counts, lower back to the start position and lower the head to the floor.

7

The Countdown Begins

Now we're just about ready to go! You know what you've got to do and why – so it's time to get prepared and let the countdown begin.

This section outlines the things you need to do before you start, based on my experience of running the 28-day plan. I have spread these tasks over five days but you can condense them into three or less days if you are in a hurry to get going. Bear in mind, though, that a little prior preparation does make a big difference in the long run and will help you get better results. In fact, there's a saying I call the five Ps: Prior Preparation Prevents Poor Performance!

FIVE DAYS TO GO: CHECK YOUR SHOES!

Put your walking shoes on the table and check them out for signs of wear and tear. Are the heels more worn down on one side? Your shoes may look in good condition from the top but your soles may tell you a different story. And are they going to give you the support you need? You don't have to fork out a fortune to get good walking shoes but your fitness and your feet are worth the investment. Any comfortable shoes will do but exercise training shoes are generally the best as they provide support and stability in the heel and forefoot, as well as a bit of lateral stability to prevent you rolling over on your ankles.

Check your socks at the same time – wearing them will help avoid blisters, and synthetic fabrics are surprisingly better for whisking away odours and perspiration! Check for signs of uneven wear on the heels or ball of the foot as this can create blisters too.

FOUR DAYS TO GO: DIG OUT YOUR WATERPROOFS

Let's have a reality check – the sun is probably not going to stay shining for you every time you go out and walk. Walking in damp weather can actually be very refreshing and enjoyable, but not if you don't have the proper kit on hand – a waterproof jacket or coat and hat. Baseball caps can be especially useful as the peak can keep the rain and wind out of your eyes. So dig out your waterproofs or borrow a friend's so you have them ready when it starts to get a little wet. Don't let this become an excuse for not doing your exercise.

Complete your fitness walking test and record your performance (see Chapter 2). Don't put this off – you will find it so rewarding, and it will give you such a sense of achievement when you finish the plan. Trust me!

THREE DAYS TO GO: PLAN YOUR FOOD SHOPPING

Read through the eating plans and Carb Curfew suppers in Chapters 3 and 5, and make yourself a list of all the foods you need for the first week. Handy containers, freezer bags and frozen fruit and vegetables can make life a lot simpler. Have a look at the shopping list, below, for help. You may also want to buy some blister pads to keep in the cupboard, just in case. If you order your shopping online, do it today so your delivery is ready to start when you are!

Shopping List

Salad greens
Canned salmon
Canned pineapple chunks in natural juice
Canned kidney beans (preferably in unsalted water)
Canned sweetcorn (preferably in unsalted, unsweetened
    water)
Jar of salsa
Cooked roast chicken

Low-fat natural yoghurt

Pre-cut and washed mixed vegetables

Fresh spinach (2 bags)

Fresh tomato or gazpacho soup from chiller cabinet

Onions

Avocado

200g packet frozen mixed seafood – mussels, cockles,
squid etc.

Eggs

Lean ham

Canned chickpeas

1 can V8 juice

Tuna canned in spring water

Canned white cannellini beans

Cherry tomatoes

Romaine or cos lettuce

Can of minestrone soup

STORE CUPBOARD ESSENTIALS

Olive oil

Balsamic vinegar

Mango chutney

Reduced-calorie French dressing

Cumin

TWO DAYS TO GO: JOT DOWN YOUR MOTIVES

Come up with five reasons why you want to lose weight: jot them down on separate pieces of paper and store them in a jar or decorative box. These motives will be there to act as reminders when your motivation fails. Keep them in a prominent place – maybe your bathroom or kitchen – so you get a little visual reminder as well. Reading reminders such as 'Fit into that pair of trousers for wedding reception', 'Lower my cholesterol and improve my health so I can play with the grandchildren', or 'Get fit so I can sign up for 5K charity event' may just give you that extra jolt to stop a cop out!

ONE DAY TO GO: CREATE A BACKUP PLAN

Map out three routes near your home, workplace or child's school of varying lengths – 10, 20, 30 and 40 metres. This will give you some options on busy days when it may not be possible to complete your walking goal. You may be short of time but creating a backup plan will stop that day becoming a disaster.

Now we really are ready to go! Remember, you will need to take your measurements on day one.

8

Your Personal Daily Charts

WEEK 1 PREVIEW

Walking Goals

Walking Novice: 15 minutes' continuous walking plus 5000 steps on your pedometer.

Walking Whiz: 30 minutes' continuous walking plus 7000 steps on your pedometer.

I will take structured exercise on these days:		**I will do my abdominal exercises on these days:**	
M	❏	M	❏
T	❏	T	❏
W	❏	W	❏
T	❏	T	❏
F	❏	F	❏
S	❏	S	❏
S	❏	S	❏

My measurements:

WEIGHT	WAIST	NAVEL	CHEST	HIPS	THIGH

This week my challenges are:

1. _____

2. _____

3. _____

4. _____

I think the week ahead will fall into the following category (circle the relevant one):

Progressive   **Maintenance**   **Damage Limitation**

DATE: _____

DAY 1

DAILY WALKING TIP: MAKE A STATEMENT

E-mail four of your friends and tell them you are starting your 28-day plan. Make the fifth e-mail to me to let me know you have started and I'll e-mail you back – e-mail me on 28daystilsuccess@joannahall.com

---

Structured Exercise: ❏

Abdominal Exercises: ❏

Steps Taken:

TIME	MEAL	ITEM	WATER TALLY	PORTION DISTORTION
	Breakfast		❑ ❑	
	Lunch		❑ ❑	
	Dinner		❑ ❑	
	Snacks		❑ ❑	
	Drinks			

DATE: _____

DAY 2

DAILY WALKING TIP: SPEED UP YOUR ARM SWING

To increase your walking pace, speed up your arm swing.
You'll find your legs will naturally speed up and fit into a
faster stride.

Structured Exercise: ❑

Abdominal Exercises: ❑

Steps Taken:

TIME	MEAL	ITEM	WATER TALLY	PORTION DISTORTION
	Breakfast		❏ ❏	
	Lunch		❏ ❏	
	Dinner		❏ ❏	
	Snacks		❏ ❏	
	Drinks			

DATE: _____

DAY 3

DAILY WALKING TIP: DIG OUT A BEAUTIFUL ROUTE

People who live near trails or walking paths are often far more physically active than those who don't. If there are none in your neighbourhood, search out your nearest National Trust park, country house and gardens, botanical garden or reservoir, then get over there before you reach Day 28 and the finish line!

Structured Exercise: ❏

Abdominal Exercises: ❏

Steps Taken:

TIME	MEAL	ITEM	WATER TALLY	PORTION DISTORTION
	Breakfast		❏ ❏	
	Lunch		❏ ❏	
	Dinner		❏ ❏	
	Snacks		❏ ❏	
	Drinks			

DATE: _____

DAY 4

DAILY WALKING TIP: BREATHE AWAY STRESS

Concentrate on breathing in through your nose and out through your mouth for at least the first few minutes of each walk. Focus on draining air into your belly first, before letting the air expand into your ribcage and chest. Deep, full breaths help relieve stress and energize your walk and your day.

Structured Exercise: ❏
Abdominal Exercises: ❏

Steps Taken:

TIME	MEAL	ITEM	WATER TALLY	PORTION DISTORTION
	Breakfast		❏ ❏	
	Lunch		❏ ❏	
	Dinner		❏ ❏	
	Snacks		❏ ❏	
	Drinks			

DATE: _____

DAY 5

DAILY WALKING TIP: STOP ACHING SHINS

This is a common problem when you try to walk faster. To get these muscles up to speed, walk on your heels for 30 seconds only (feet flexed and toes pointing towards the sky). Repeat three times during your walk on two or three days a week.

Structured Exercise: ❏

Abdominal Exercises: ❏

Steps Taken:

TIME	MEAL	ITEM	WATER TALLY	PORTION DISTORTION
	Breakfast		❑ ❑	
	Lunch		❑ ❑	
	Dinner		❑ ❑	
	Snacks		❑ ❑	
	Drinks			

DATE: _____

DAY 6

DAILY WALKING TIP: VISUALIZE FULL GLASSES

To help minimize any shin or back pain, imagine you have a full cup of water balanced on each hip as you walk. Pulling in your tummy muscles and lifting up out of your hips will not only improve your posture and reduce backache but you'll instantly look better too.

Structured Exercise: ❑

Abdominal Exercises: ❑

Steps Taken:

TIME	MEAL	ITEM	WATER TALLY	PORTION DISTORTION
	Breakfast		❏ ❏	
	Lunch		❏ ❏	
	Dinner		❏ ❏	
	Snacks		❏ ❏	
	Drinks			

DATE: _____

DAY 7

DAILY WALKING TIP: REDUCE THE IMPACT

If you have a choice of walking on a concrete pavement or an asphalt road, choose the latter because it is softer. If the road slants towards the kerb, reverse the direction you walk every couple of days to avoid injuries resulting from walking on uneven surfaces.

Structured Exercise: ❏

Abdominal Exercises: ❏

Steps Taken:

TIME	MEAL	ITEM	WATER TALLY	PORTION DISTORTION
	Breakfast		❑ ❑	
	Lunch		❑ ❑	
	Dinner		❑ ❑	
	Snacks		❑ ❑	
	Drinks			

WEEK 1 REVIEW

I took structured exercise on the following days:

M ☐

T ☐

W ☐

T ☐

F ☐

S ☐

S ☐

My measurements:

WEIGHT	WAIST	NAVEL	CHEST	HIPS	THIGH

I did my abdominal exercises on these days:

M ☐

T ☐

W ☐

T ☐

F ☐

S ☐

S ☐

On reflection my week fell into the following category (circle the relevant one):

Progressive   **Maintenance**   **Damage Limitation**

WEEK 2 PREVIEW

Walking Goals

Walking Novice: 20 minutes' continuous walking plus 8000 steps on your pedometer.

Walking Whiz: 40 minutes' continuous walking plus 9000 steps on your pedometer.

I will take structured exercise on these days:

M ❑

T ❑

W ❑

T ❑

F ❑

S ❑

S ❑

I will do my abdominal exercises on these days:

M   ❑

T   ❑

W   ❑

T   ❑

F   ❑

S   ❑

S   ❑

This week my challenges are:

1. _____

2. _____

3. _____

4. _____

I think the week ahead will fall into the following category (circle the relevant one):

Progressive   **Maintenance**   **Damage Limitation**

DATE: _____

DAY 8

DAILY WALKING TIP: BREATHING

To avoid snatching your breaths and getting a stitch, focus on your breathing technique. Try to take a breath in on four counts or strides, and take four strides or counts to breathe out.

Structured Exercise: ❑

Abdominal Exercises: ❑

Steps Taken:

TIME	MEAL	ITEM	WATER TALLY	PORTION DISTORTION
	Breakfast		❏ ❏	
	Lunch		❏ ❏	
	Dinner		❏ ❏	
	Snacks		❏ ❏	
	Drinks			

DATE: _____

DAY 9

DAILY WALKING TIP: FIND A TUNE

Why not listen to an up-tempo favourite tune as you walk today? It can get you walking faster.

Structured Exercise: ❑

Abdominal Exercises: ❑

Steps Taken:

TIME	MEAL	ITEM	WATER TALLY	PORTION DISTORTION
	Breakfast		❏ ❏	
	Lunch		❏ ❏	
	Dinner		❏ ❏	
	Snacks		❏ ❏	
	Drinks			

DATE: _____

DAY 10

DAILY WALKING TIP: WEAR A BELT TO GET A BETTER BOTTOM

Believe it or not, wearing a belt will help you get a better backside. Put on a snugly fitting belt and pull in your abdominals so you create a space between the belt and the belly. This helps flatten your tummy and stabilize your pelvis, which then improves the toning effects on your bottom with each walking stride!

Structured Exercise: ❏

Abdominal Exercises: ❏

Steps Taken:

TIME	MEAL	ITEM	WATER TALLY	PORTION DISTORTION
	Breakfast		❑ ❑	
	Lunch		❑ ❑	
	Dinner		❑ ❑	
	Snacks		❑ ❑	
	Drinks			

DATE: _____

DAY 11

DAILY WALKING TIP: GET OUT OF A SLUMP

To stand up straight, bend your left arm behind your waist and grab your right arm at the elbow. This simple movement pulls your shoulders back and down. Hold for about 10 seconds and then switch arms. Do this two or three times during each walk.

Structured Exercise: ❏

Abdominal Exercises: ❏

Steps Taken:

TIME	MEAL	ITEM	WATER TALLY	PORTION DISTORTION
	Breakfast		❑ ❑	
	Lunch		❑ ❑	
	Dinner		❑ ❑	
	Snacks		❑ ❑	
	Drinks			

DATE: _____

DAY 12

DAILY WALKING TIP: KEEP YOUR HANDS FREE

You can stash away everything you need, like keys, money and mobile phone, in a stylish bum bag. Keeping your hands free will help your walking technique and allow you to run some errands as you hit your walking target.

Structured Exercise: ❑

Abdominal Exercises: ❑

Steps Taken:

TIME	MEAL	ITEM	WATER TALLY	PORTION DISTORTION
	Breakfast		❑ ❑	
	Lunch		❑ ❑	
	Dinner		❑ ❑	
	Snacks		❑ ❑	
	Drinks			

DATE: _____

DAY 13

DAILY WALKING TIP: DON'T USE WEIGHTS

Don't be fooled into thinking that holding hand weights while walking will make your workout harder and help you burn more calories. Studies show that for your body to achieve any additional calorie expenditure from carrying hand weights as you walk, you need to hold a minimum of 3 pounds in each hand. This is actually quite a load, and the small additional increase in calorie burn is outweighed by the potential strain at the shoulder joint. Adding inclines and hills into your walk is a much more efficient way to burn extra calories (see tip for Day 17).

Structured Exercise: ❑

Abdominal Exercises: ❑

Steps Taken:

TIME	MEAL	ITEM	WATER TALLY	PORTION DISTORTION
	Breakfast		❏ ❏	
	Lunch		❏ ❏	
	Dinner		❏ ❏	
	Snacks		❏ ❏	
	Drinks			

DATE: _____

DAY 14

DAILY WALKING TIP: TAKE A HALF-TIME BREAK

You're off the hook today: walk only half of the recommended time, but do it at a faster pace than usual. This is a great way to fit in a full workout when your schedule is tight. You can burn the same number of calories whether you walk for 40 minutes at 3 mph or 20 minutes at 4 mph.

Structured Exercise: ❏

Abdominal Exercises: ❏

Steps Taken:

TIME	MEAL	ITEM	WATER TALLY	PORTION DISTORTION
	Breakfast		❏ ❏	
	Lunch		❏ ❏	
	Dinner		❏ ❏	
	Snacks		❏ ❏	
	Drinks			

WEEK 2 REVIEW

I took structured exercise on the following days:

M ☐

T ☐

W ☐

T ☐

F ☐

S ☐

S ☐

My measurements:

WEIGHT	WAIST	NAVEL	CHEST	HIPS	THIGH

I did my abdominal exercises on these days:

M ☐

T ☐

W ☐

T ☐

F ☐

S ☐

S ☐

On reflection my week fell into the following category (circle the relevant one):

Progressive   **Maintenance**   **Damage Limitation**

WEEK 3 PREVIEW

Walking Goals

Walking Novice: 25 minutes' continuous walking plus 9000 steps on your pedometer.

Walking Whiz: 45 minutes' continuous walking per day or two bouts of continuous walking totalling 45 minutes plus 9000 steps on your pedometer.

I will take structured exercise on these days:

M ☐

T ☐

W ☐

T ☐

F ☐

S ☐

S ☐

I will do my abdominal exercises on these days:

M ☐

T ☐

W ☐

T ☐

F ☐

S ☐

S ☐

This week my challenges are:

1. _____

2. _____

3. _____

4. _____

I think the week ahead will fall into the following category
(circle the relevant one):

Progressive   **Maintenance**   **Damage
                                                  Limitation**

DATE: _____

DAY 15

DAILY WALKING TIP: PLAY WITH YOUR BREAK POINT

You can raise your exercise calorie burn by playing with your break point. To find it, walk as fast as you can, speeding up your arm swing will naturally increase your leg stride. Make sure you maintain good technique and try to increase your walking pace progressively until you feel you are just about to break into a jog. This is your break point. Walking at this pace will feel slightly uncomfortable and difficult so use it to find your optimum walking pace and to boost your calorie burn on some of your structured walking sessions. Try walking for 15 seconds at your break point pace every three minutes.

Structured Exercise: ❑

Abdominal Exercises: ❑

Steps Taken:

TIME	MEAL	ITEM	WATER TALLY	PORTION DISTORTION
	Breakfast		❑ ❑	
	Lunch		❑ ❑	
	Dinner		❑ ❑	
	Snacks		❑ ❑	
	Drinks			

DATE: _____

DAY 16

DAILY WALKING TIP: REVIEW YOUR FITNESS WALKING TEST

Remember your fitness walking test route (see Chapter 2)? Today go and have a practice walk on it as part of your workout.

Structured Exercise: ❏

Abdominal Exercises: ❏

Steps Taken:

TIME	MEAL	ITEM	WATER TALLY	PORTION DISTORTION
	Breakfast		❏ ❏	
	Lunch		❏ ❏	
	Dinner		❏ ❏	
	Snacks		❏ ❏	
	Drinks			

DATE: _____

DAY 17

DAILY WALKING TIP: RAISE YOUR INCLINE

Start climbing – hill walking burns up to 60 per cent more calories than walking at the same pace on level ground, and it's great for firming your backside. If you are struggling to find a route with an incline, why not go to your local leisure centre or gym and jump on a tread-mill? It's easy to raise the incline on these machines.

Structured Exercise: ❏
Abdominal Exercises: ❏

Steps Taken:

TIME	MEAL	ITEM	WATER TALLY	PORTION DISTORTION
	Breakfast		❑ ❑	
	Lunch		❑ ❑	
	Dinner		❑ ❑	
	Snacks		❑ ❑	
	Drinks			

DATE: _____

DAY 18

DAILY WALKING TIP: CHANGE YOUR WALKING RHYTHM

Changing the rhythm of your walk can boost your energy. Instead of the usual two-count or four-count step (left right, left right), count in threes. Chant a positive mantra, such as "Yes I can!"

Structured Exercise: ❑

Abdominal Exercises: ❑

Steps Taken:

TIME	MEAL	ITEM	WATER TALLY	PORTION DISTORTION
	Breakfast		❏ ❏	
	Lunch		❏ ❏	
	Dinner		❏ ❏	
	Snacks		❏ ❏	
	Drinks			

DATE: _____

DAY 19

DAILY WALKING TIP: ADD WALKING LUNGES

Add eight lunges after each 10 minutes of walking this week. If you are a walking novice, introduce four lunges every five minutes. Stand in neutral position. Take a large step back with one leg, ensuring the front knee stays over the ankle and is not turned in. The extended leg should have a slight bend at the knee, while the rear heel should be off the ground. Lunge by bending your rear leg so that the knee comes close to the ground. Draw up through your abdominals as you lift your leg back to the start position.

Structured Exercise: ❏

Abdominal Exercises: ❏

Steps Taken:

TIME	MEAL	ITEM	WATER TALLY	PORTION DISTORTION
	Breakfast		❑ ❑	
	Lunch		❑ ❑	
	Dinner		❑ ❑	
	Snacks		❑ ❑	
	Drinks			

DATE: _____

DAY 20

DAILY WALKING TIP: HOP, SKIP AND JUMP!

To improve balance and co-ordination, build bone and burn fat faster, add some play to your walk. If you walk in a group, break out in a park and play a few minutes of 'It' or 'Tag'! Hop on and off curbs, zigzag in and out of trees, attack any sloping terrain head on and bunny hop across path edges. Do these moves carefully so you don't trip.

Structured Exercise: ❑

Abdominal Exercises: ❑

Steps Taken:

TIME	MEAL	ITEM	WATER TALLY	PORTION DISTORTION
	Breakfast		❑ ❑	
	Lunch		❑ ❑	
	Dinner		❑ ❑	
	Snacks		❑ ❑	
	Drinks			

DATE: _____

DAY 21

DAILY WALKING TIP: WIGGLE YOUR HIPS

Add a race-walking hip swivel to increase speed, trim your waistline and burn more calories. Walk slowly, crossing your feet slightly in front of you so one hip rotates forward while the other goes back. Once you get the hang of it, pick up your pace and try it without crossing your feet.

Structured Exercise: ❑

Abdominal Exercises: ❑

Steps Taken:

TIME	MEAL	ITEM	WATER TALLY	PORTION DISTORTION
	Breakfast		❏ ❏	
	Lunch		❏ ❏	
	Dinner		❏ ❏	
	Snacks		❏ ❏	
	Drinks			

WEEK 3 REVIEW

I took structured exercise on the following days:

M   ☐

T   ☐

W   ☐

T   ☐

F   ☐

S   ☐

S   ☐

My measurements:

WEIGHT	WAIST	NAVEL	CHEST	HIPS	THIGH

I did my abdominal exercises on these days:

M ☐

T ☐

W ☐

T ☐

F ☐

S ☐

S ☐

On reflection my week fell into the following category (circle the relevant one):

Progressive   **Maintenance**   **Damage Limitation**

WEEK 4 PREVIEW

Walking Goals

Walking Novice: 30 minutes' continuous walking plus 10,000 steps on your pedometer.

Walking Whiz: 50 minutes' continuous walking each day plus 10,000 steps on your pedometer.

I will take structured exercise on these days:

M ❏

T ❏

W ❏

T ❏

F ❏

S ❏

S ❏

I will do my abdominal exercises on these days:

M ☐

T ☐

W ☐

T ☐

F ☐

S ☐

S ☐

This week my challenges are:

1. _____

2. _____

3. _____

4. _____

I think the week ahead will fall into the following category (circle the relevant one):

Progressive   **Maintenance**   **Damage Limitation**

DATE: _____

DAY 22

DAILY WALKING TIP: GO FOR A MOONWALK

Put on some reflective clothing, grab your partner or a friend and a flashlight and head out on a night walk. Night noises, a starry night sky and even window shopping can give a refreshing spark to a familiar route. But do remember to walk in a safe area.

Structured Exercise: ❑

Abdominal Exercises: ❑

Steps Taken:

TIME	MEAL	ITEM	WATER TALLY	PORTION DISTORTION
	Breakfast		❏ ❏	
	Lunch		❏ ❏	
	Dinner		❏ ❏	
	Snacks		❏ ❏	
	Drinks			

DATE: _____

DAY 23

DAILY WALKING TIP: INVEST IN A WEIGHTED VEST

Walking with hand weights can strain your shoulders. A safer way to up your intensity is a weighted vest that distributes the extra pounds evenly.

Structured Exercise: ❑

Abdominal Exercises: ❑

Steps Taken:

TIME	MEAL	ITEM	WATER TALLY	PORTION DISTORTION
	Breakfast		❑ ❑	
	Lunch		❑ ❑	
	Dinner		❑ ❑	
	Snacks		❑ ❑	
	Drinks			

DATE: _____

DAY 24

DAILY WALKING TIP: KEEP UP THE GOOD WORK!

For a double dose of feel-good vibes, lend your feet to a cause. Training for and completing a charity walk with a large group of people is exhilarating. Knowing you are ticking off a good deed in the process makes your success all the more enjoyable. And committing to an event will help you keep up your walking programme.

Structured Exercise: ❏

Abdominal Exercises: ❏

Steps Taken:

TIME	MEAL	ITEM	WATER TALLY	PORTION DISTORTION
	Breakfast		❑	
			❑	
	Lunch		❑	
			❑	
	Dinner		❑	
			❑	
	Snacks		❑	
			❑	
	Drinks			

DATE: _____

DAY 25

DAILY WALKING TIP: BACK DOWN

Walk briskly up a hill or stairs, then slowly go down backwards to stretch the calves, hamstrings and go easy on your knees. Do be careful and watch where you are going.

Structured Exercise: ❑

Abdominal Exercises: ❑

Steps Taken:

TIME	MEAL	ITEM	WATER TALLY	PORTION DISTORTION
	Breakfast		❏ ❏	
	Lunch		❏ ❏	
	Dinner		❏ ❏	
	Snacks		❏ ❏	
	Drinks			

DATE: _____

DAY 26

DAILY WALKING TIP: HAVE A COFFEE BREAK

Split your walk in two today. Plan a route so you walk to a coffee shop and have a quick coffee and a chat with a friend before completing the second half of your walk.

Structured Exercise: ❏

Abdominal Exercises: ❏

Steps Taken:

TIME	MEAL	ITEM	WATER TALLY	PORTION DISTORTION
	Breakfast		❏ ❏	
	Lunch		❏ ❏	
	Dinner		❏ ❏	
	Snacks		❏ ❏	
	Drinks			

DATE: _____

DAY 27

DAILY WALKING TIP: HIT THE BEACH!

Walking in soft sand boosts your calorie burn by 20–50 per cent, and it will wake up leg muscles you never knew you had.

Structured Exercise: ❏

Abdominal Exercises: ❏

Steps Taken:

TIME	MEAL	ITEM	WATER TALLY	PORTION DISTORTION
	Breakfast		❏ ❏	
	Lunch		❏ ❏	
	Dinner		❏ ❏	
	Snacks		❏ ❏	
	Drinks			

DATE: _____

DAY 28

**DAILY WALKING TIP: CONGRATULATIONS!
YOU'VE MADE IT!!**

E-mail the four friends you contacted at the start of your
28-day programme and me (28daystilsuccess@joanna-
hall.com) to tell them (and me!) you have completed
your challenge.

Structured Exercise: ❏

Abdominal Exercises: ❏

Steps Taken:

TIME	MEAL	ITEM	WATER TALLY	PORTION DISTORTION
	Breakfast		❏ ❏	
	Lunch		❏ ❏	
	Dinner		❏ ❏	
	Snacks		❏ ❏	
	Drinks			

WEEK 4 REVIEW

I took structured exercise on the following days:

M   ❑

T   ❑

W   ❑

T   ❑

F   ❑

S   ❑

S   ❑

My measurements:

WEIGHT	WAIST	NAVEL	CHEST	HIPS	THIGH

I did my abdominal exercises on these days:

M   ❑

T   ❑

W   ❑

T   ❑

F   ❑

S   ❑

S   ❑

On reflection my week fell into the following category (circle the relevant one):

Progressive   **Maintenance**   **Damage Limitation**

28-DAY REVIEW

I did my abdominal exercises on this many days:

_____

My final measurements:

WEIGHT	WAIST	NAVEL	CHEST	HIPS	THIGH

My starting measurements:

WEIGHT	WAIST	NAVEL	CHEST	HIPS	THIGH

Subtracting final from starting measurements, I have lost:

WEIGHT	WAIST	NAVEL	CHEST	HIPS	THIGH

On reflection my month was:
(circle one)

Inspiring!

Congratulations! You have done a great job – and I hope you enjoyed your 28-day plan. Give yourself a pat on the back!

Be active,

Joanna

9

The Step Trade Offs

If you really can't resist the odd snack, then Step Trade Offs are the answer. These are a guide to the number of steps you will need to take to burn off those calories. Please bear in mind that this is a guideline only, as portion sizes, calorie content and walking speed are all variable.

The idea is simple – applying the trade-off means you don't have to deprive yourself of your favourite foods. If you fancy a packet of crisps, fine, go ahead have them. Just look them up on the list below and see how many extra steps you'll need to take. Remember: counting steps to keep your energy gap in the right direction should be a tool and not an obsession.

So, for example:

6 chocolate biscuits OR
1 McDonald's cheeseburger OR
3 large oranges

contain 300 calories, and you need to take a 3-mile brisk walk or 6,000 steps on your pedometer to burn them off.

Remember: any additional physical activity goes towards justifying that snack and keeping your energy gap in balance.

So follow the step trade-off chart on page 201 to see how you can still enjoy some of the snacks you may be tempted to splurge on. You might be surprised at the number of steps you will need to burn off that snack indulgence! This is not about saying you can *never* have snacks, but this simple trade-off can quickly and easily put things in perspective, as well as encouraging you to increase your overall level of physical activity.

FOOD ITEM	CALORIES	NUMBER OF PEDOMETER STEPS
1 milk chocolate digestive biscuit	86	2,150
1 Golden Crunch Cream biscuit	66	1,650
1 bagel (standard size)	230	5,750
5cm-long garlic ciabatta bread	200	5,000
1 plain naan bread	294	7,350
1 chocolate brownie cake	328	8,200
2 chocolate cookies	174	4,350
1 pecan Danish pastry	287	7,175
1 jam doughnut	324	8,100
1 shop-bought blueberry muffin	438	10,950
1 pain au chocolat	235	5,875
1 McDonald's Big Breakfast	591	14,775
1 KFC Fillet Towermeal Burger	656	16,400
1 Burger King Whopper with mayo	678	16,950
8 Pizza Express mini dough balls	200	5,000
1 McDonald's Creme Egg McFlurry	390	9,750
1 Pizza Express American Hot Pizza	788	19,700
1 Pizza Hut Margherita Stuffed Crust Original	330	8,250
1 McDonald's Hot Fudge Sundae	352	8,800

1 Cod Fish & Chips ready-meal (Waitrose)	849	21,225
1 sushi fish box (large, Tesco)	423	10,575
1 Cornish pasty (Pork Farms)	673	16,825
1 Melton Mowbray pork pie (Tesco)	679	16,975
2 thick pork & beef sausages	330	8,250
1 large sausage roll (Ginsters)	753	18,825
1 Scotch egg (Asda)	286	7,150
1 individual quiche Lorraine (Tesco)	262	6,550
1 large Yorkshire pudding (Auntie Bessie's)	104	2,600
1 Tuna Melt sandwich (Marks & Spencer)	621	15,525
1 ready-made cheese sandwich (Asda)	618	15,450
1 whole Terry's Milk Chocolate Orange	928	23,200
1 Cadbury's Double Decker bar	237	5,925
1 packet Milky Haribo sweet mix (175g)	644	16,100
1 large can Heinz baked beans	303	7,575
1 Sweet & Sour Chicken with Rice ready-meal (Asda)	440	11,000
1 Chicken Tikka Masala ready-meal (Sainsbury's)	848	21,200

1 Ham & Mushroom Tagliatelle ready-meal (Sainsbury's)	486	12,150
1 shop-bought Tuna & Sweetcorn Jacket Potato (Somerfield)	333	8,325
Cheese & Bacon Potato Skins (Tesco)	241	6,025
1 McDonald's chocolate milkshake (regular)	403	10,075
1 King Size Salted French Fries (Burger King)	539	13,475
1 Strawberries & Banana Smoothie (Innocent)	118	2,950
1 bottle Original Lucozade (small/345ml)	252	6,300
1 can Fanta Lemon drink	165	4,125
1 coffee latte (Pret A Manger)	194	4,850
1 bag caramel Snack-a-Jacks	140	3,500
1 carton salted popcorn (Blockbuster)	121	3,025
1 small bag salt & vinegar crisps (Walkers)	186	4,650
3 roast potatoes	280	7,000

10

Carb Curfew Recipes

In devising these recipes I worked with Louise Shaxson of www.whoscomingtodinner.com

MEAT DISHES

Sausages and Lentils with a Beetroot and Walnut Salad

Serves 2, with leftovers

This is a lovely filling dish with glorious colours and textures. Make sure you use good-quality butcher's sausages which have a very high percentage of meat and less fat. You must use dark-green (Puy) lentils for this as they taste fabulous and hold together well when you cook them. They are widely available, but you might have to look in the specialist sections of the supermarket. Any leftovers are delicious the next day: mix the sliced cold sausages with the lentils and beetroot for a simple one-dish lunch that tastes as good cold as it does hot.

Prep time: 5 minutes
Cooking time: 40 minutes

250g Puy lentils

1 wine glass of red wine (optional)

3 sprigs rosemary

4 good-quality sausages (such as Cumberland:
    about 50g per sausage)

200g cooked beetroot (not pickled)

3 tbsp (30g) chopped walnuts

Salt and pepper to taste

1 tbsp walnut oil

4 tbsp olive oil

2 tbsp red wine vinegar (or to taste)

Put the lentils in a heavy-bottomed pan with a lid. Add the wine if using, 350ml water and 2 sprigs of rosemary, bring to the boil and then lower the heat and simmer gently, with the lid on, for 30 minutes. Check after 20 minutes to make sure the lentils aren't drying out, adding more water if needed. They should be 'al dente' when done.

While the lentils are cooking, heat the grill and cook the sausages. These are best done slowly, so put the grill on a low shelf and take your time over them.

While the lentils and sausages are cooking, chop the beetroot into bite-sized chunks. Add the walnuts, 1 sprig of rosemary, a little salt and pepper and the walnut oil and stir to coat. Taste and correct the seasoning.

When the lentils are done, remove them from the heat and take out the rosemary sprigs. Add 1 tsp of salt, a few grindings of black pepper, 2 tbsp olive oil and the red wine vinegar. Stir gently, check the taste, and leave with the lid on until you are ready to serve. Place a mound of lentils on the plate, top with the sausages and spread the beetroot and walnut salad around the sides.

Per serving:

Carbs	40.8g
Proteins	14.15g
Fat	22.85g
Calories	449 (with wine) or 398 (without)

Grilled Lamb Chops with Flageolet Beans and Rosemary-roasted Cherry Tomatoes

Serves 2

Based on a classic French dish, this is delicious and very filling. The roasted cherry tomatoes have a lovely flavour and look great on the plate.

Prep time: 10 minutes
Cooking time: 30 minutes

2 lamb chops, fat removed (150g per chop)

For the tomatoes:
250g ripe cherry tomatoes
1 sprig rosemary
4 cloves garlic, unpeeled
1 tbsp olive oil
1 tbsp balsamic vinegar
½ tsp sugar
½ tsp salt

For the flageolets:

1 x 410g can flageolet beans, drained and rinsed in
   cold water

1 shallot, peeled and very finely chopped

1 clove garlic, crushed

2 tbsp low-fat plain yoghurt

Salt and black pepper

1 tbsp pumpkin seed oil

4 sprigs rosemary (to garnish)

Remove the lamb chops from the fridge so they are at room temperature before you cook them. Start by roasting the cherry tomatoes: preheat the oven to 200°C/400°F/Gas Mark 6. Lay the tomatoes in an oven-proof serving dish and prick each one with the point of a sharp knife. Add a sprig of rosemary and the unpeeled garlic cloves and toss it all together with the olive oil, balsamic vinegar, sugar and salt. Roast in the middle of the oven for 25 minutes.

When the tomatoes are cooked, remove and leave to one side: they actually taste better if they're not too hot. Preheat the grill and grill the lamb for about 4 minutes each side (depending on how thick the chops are). When they are almost done, turn off the grill and leave the chops to rest on a low shelf in the oven with the door slightly open. This helps the meat to relax. While the lamb is grilling, place the flageolet beans, shallot and garlic into another saucepan and add 3 tbsp cold water. Cook over a medium heat until the shallot is soft.

Stir the yoghurt into the warmed beans and pour them onto the plates. Season the beans and drizzle with the pumpkin seed oil, then lay the lamb chops on the side. Add the roasted cherry tomatoes with their juices to the plate, and garnish each plate with a sprig of rosemary.

Per serving:

Carbs	25.0g
Proteins	37.5g
Fat	16.7g
Calories	389

Pork Chops with Cannellini Beans in a Tomato and Mushroom Sauce

Serves 2

This is a delicious one-pot dish, full of warmth.

Prep time: 15 minutes
Cooking time: 30 minutes

For the sauce:
10g dried porcini mushrooms
1 x 400g can chopped plum tomatoes
2 medium-sized fresh tomatoes, chopped into smallish chunks
1 shallot, finely chopped
1 stick celery, finely chopped

1 tbsp olive oil or cooking oil spray
2 pork chops, fat removed: 125g per portion
100g sliced mushrooms
1 x 410g can cannellini beans, drained and rinsed in
    cold water
3 tbsp semi-skimmed milk
Salt and pepper
100g green beans, topped and tailed
15g flat-leaf parsley, finely chopped

First, make the sauce. Soak the porcini in 125ml water for 20 minutes, then drain and chop finely. Don't throw away the soaking liquid, but put it in a medium-sized saucepan with the tinned tomatoes, fresh tomatoes, shallot, celery and chopped porcini. Bring to the boil and simmer for a few minutes.

Add the oil to a non-stick frying pan and fry the pork chops over a high heat until nicely browned on both sides. Turn the heat down and add the tomato and porcini sauce. Put the lid on tightly and simmer gently for 30 minutes.

Ten minutes before serving, gently stir the sliced mushrooms, cannellini beans and milk into the sauce around the pork chops. Taste and add salt and pepper if you need to. Reheat and simmer gently while you deal with the green beans.

Put the green beans into a microwave-proof bowl with 2 tbsp cold water. Cover tightly with clingfilm and microwave on high for 3 minutes. Drain the beans before serving, and sprinkle the parsley over the top of the pork as a garnish.

Per serving:

Carbs	28.5g
Proteins	32.35g
Fat	7.2g
Calories	354

Mixed Bean Salad with Parma Ham and Rocket

Serves 2

Serve this salad at room temperature to really get the flavours. It keeps well in the fridge but you can refresh it by adding a few more shredded basil leaves and a little more vinegar. The pumpkin seeds in the rocket salad give a delicious crunch.

Prep time: 10 minutes
Cooking time: none

1 x 410g can mixed bean salad, drained and rinsed
    (or substitute a can of cannellini beans)
3 large ripe tomatoes (200g), chopped into bite-sized chunks
15 black Greek olives (40g), drained from a can in brine
1 shallot, finely chopped and rinsed with cold water
30g fresh Parmesan, finely grated
15g (a small handful) flat-leaf parsley, finely chopped
6 fresh basil leaves, torn into strips
4 slices Parma ham (100g)
1 bag rocket leaves (100g), or rocket/spinach/watercress
    salad, washed and drained
2 tbsp (10g) pumpkin seeds

Dressing:

2 tbsp extra-virgin olive oil

2 tbsp white wine vinegar

2 tbsp pesto sauce

1 small clove garlic, minced or grated

Salt and pepper to taste

Mix the beans, tomatoes, olives, chopped shallot, Parmesan and parsley together in a large bowl. Combine the dressing ingredients in a screw-top jar and shake vigorously. Pour two-thirds of the dressing over the salad and mix well, leaving to stand for 10 minutes before eating so the flavours can meld together. Taste and correct for salt, pesto, vinegar, garlic, or whatever other flavour you need.

Just before serving, mix the torn basil leaves into the bean salad. Arrange the Parma ham on the plate and pile some of the dressed bean salad on the side. Toss the rocket leaves or the bag of green salad with the pumpkin seeds and the rest of the dressing, and pile onto the plate.

Per serving:

Carbs	24.1g
Proteins	29.0g
Fat	23.7g
Calories	459

Pork Chops with Baked Pears, Butternut Squash and Mint Vinaigrette

Serves 2

This was inspired by a Jamie Oliver dish. It's very simple, but with lots of colour and flavour. It would work very well at a dinner party.

Prep time: 10 minutes
Cooking time: 30 minutes

2 pork chops: 125g per portion, fat removed (loin chops, chump chops or leg steaks work well)
30 mint leaves (a good big handful), finely chopped
2 sprigs rosemary, leaves removed and very finely chopped
2 tbsp white wine vinegar
3 tbsp olive oil
2 tbsp water
½ tsp salt
2 pears, not too ripe
200g butternut squash

Take the pork chops out of the fridge while you prepare the rest of the ingredients: meat cooks so much
better at room temperature. Trim them of as much
fat as you can. Preheat the oven to 200°C/400°F/Gas
Mark 6.

Mix the mint leaves, half the rosemary, the vinegar,
olive oil, water and salt in a small bowl. Smear about
a tablespoonful over each chop and leave to marinade.
Quarter and core the pears, then chop each piece in
half. Cut the butternut squash into half-inch cubes:
you don't even need to remove the skin as it softens
wonderfully when you cook it.

Place the cubed pears and squash on a baking tray,
sprinkle with the remaining chopped rosemary and
put in the middle of the oven for 10 minutes: you
don't need any oil as their natural sugars will help give
them that roasted taste. Add the pork chops to the tray
and return to the oven for another 15–20 minutes,
depending on the thickness of the chops. Remove the
chops to your plates, and toss the roasted vegetables
with the rest of the mint vinaigrette before piling
them up at the side. Enjoy!

Per serving:

Carbs	17.4g
Proteins	22.5g
Fat	10.5g
Calories	299

Ham with Broad Beans in a Simple Parsley Sauce

Serves 2

This is a simple, low-fat way of serving ham in a parsley sauce. The sweetness of the broad beans is delicious with the ham, so even if you think you don't like them, you will!

Prep time: 2 minutes
Cooking time: 3 minutes

200g frozen baby broad beans
30g flat-leaf parsley, leaves removed and finely
   chopped
2 tsp olive oil
125ml (3 tbsp) low-fat plain yoghurt
Several good grindings of black pepper
½ tsp salt
2 good thick slices of roast ham, with the fat removed
   (125g per portion)

Put the frozen broad beans and the chopped parsley into a microwave-proof bowl, add a few tablespoons of cold water and cover with clingfilm. Cook on high for 3 minutes then drain, retaining as much of the parsley as you can. Stir the olive oil and yoghurt into the beans, and add the black pepper. You may want to return the beans to the microwave to reheat (medium heat for 1 minute) but don't overcook them. Remember that the ham will be very salty, so don't add salt until you've tasted them all together.

Serve the ham with the beans on the side.

Per serving:

Carbs	15.45g
Proteins	40.45g
Fat	5.5g
Calories	334

Griddled Chicken Breast with Roasted Vegetable Ratatouille

Serves 2

This is an incredibly simple meal with huge tastes. It makes a great midweek supper and is smart enough to impress guests at a dinner party. You could easily serve the ratatouille with steak, grilled white fish or barbecued lamb. You need your largest baking tray so that the vegetables lie in a single layer and roast properly.

Prep time: 10 minutes
Cooking time: 30 minutes

2 skinless chicken breasts, 150g each
1 medium aubergine (100g)
2 courgettes (200g)
2 red peppers (100g)
2 medium onions (200g)
3 cloves garlic
200g cherry or baby plum tomatoes
3 tbsp olive oil
1 sprig rosemary
125ml of your favourite tomato-based pasta sauce
Salt and pepper to taste

For the marinade:

1 clove garlic

1 sprig rosemary

125ml white wine

1 tbsp olive oil

If you have time, marinade the chicken breasts before you make the ratatouille. Chop the garlic and rosemary roughly, add the wine and olive oil and pour over the chicken breasts. Cover with clingfilm and set aside at room temperature.

Heat the oven to 200°C/400°F/Gas Mark 6. Top and tail the aubergine and courgettes, deseed the peppers, and peel, top and tail the onions. Cut them all into bite-sized pieces. Cut the bottom off the garlic but don't peel it, and then place all the vegetables (except the rosemary) onto the baking tray. Mix them all together with 2 tbsp olive oil, either with your hands or a wooden spoon, and spread them out evenly. Roast the vegetables in the top of the oven for about 40 minutes. When done, remove them from the oven, fish out the garlic and slip off its skin. Mash the roasted garlic with the pasta sauce in a saucepan, then add the rest of the roasted vegetables to the same pan. Add the rosemary and stir: you may need to add a little more pasta sauce to bind it together. Reheat very gently while you cook the chicken breasts.

Heat a ridged griddle pan if you have one, or use a regular frying pan. When it is very hot, drain much of the marinade from the chicken breasts and cook for about 5 minutes on each side until done, basting with the marinade as you go. Serve a mound of ratatouille on each plate, topped with a chicken breast.

Per serving:

Carbs	21.95g
Proteins	52.15g
Fat	14.2g
Calories	147

FISH DISHES

Summer Salad of Poached Salmon with Spinach and Mangetout and Minty Yoghurt Dressing

Serves 2

You can poach the salmon steaks yourself, or you can buy ready-poached salmon flakes which you could toss together with the spinach and mint to make a one-dish salad. The whole mint leaves give a great fresh taste.

Prep time: 5 minutes
Cooking time: 15 minutes

Either 2 salmon steaks (125g per portion) and 1 lemon
   or 250g poached salmon flakes
1 pack baby spinach leaves
1 large handful (50g) mangetout or sugar snap peas
15g fresh mint (a good handful)
4 tbsp low-fat mayonnaise
200ml plain yoghurt
Salt to taste

If you are poaching the salmon yourself, put the steaks into a pan of cold water with the juice of 1 lemon, and bring slowly to the boil. Simmer gently for 5 minutes, and then turn off the heat and leave them to cool naturally. They will be lovely and moist.

Wash the spinach and the mangetout or sugar snap peas, and chop them roughly. Strip the mint leaves from their stems and set aside about 20: these will go into the salad whole. Put the rest of the mint, the mayonnaise, yoghurt and the juice of half the lemon into the food processor and blend until smooth. Taste and correct for salt and/or lemon: remember that a squeeze of lemon juice is a good substitute for salt, so add the lemon first and then taste to see if you need more salt.

Toss the spinach and mangetout together and lay on a plate. Place the salmon on top (or sprinkle the salmon flakes over the top of the salad) before drizzling the green dressing over it all.

Per serving:

Carbs	10.65g
Proteins	29.1g
Fat	19.1g
Calories	331

Baked Trout with Peas and Pesto

Serves 2

This is the simplest of suppers, but quite delicious. Trout fillets cook faster, but you might find you get more flavour with the whole fish. Peas with pesto are a great alternative to peas with mint; try them with grilled lamb chops as well.

Prep time: 5 minutes

Cooking time: 20 minutes (less if you are using trout fillets)

4 trout fillets (skin on: 125g per portion) or 2 whole
    trout, cleaned and washed

1 lemon, sliced

300g frozen peas

2 tbsp pesto

A few fresh basil leaves, roughly torn or chopped

Spray a little oil over a sheet of tinfoil to stop the trout sticking to it. Put the plates to warm in the oven.

If you have whole trout, preheat the oven to 200°C/400°F/Gas Mark 6. Put a few slices of lemon inside the trout and lay it on the baking sheet. Bake the trout, uncovered, for 15–20 minutes until the skin is crispy and a skewer goes through with no resistance.

If *you have* trout *fillets*, preheat the grill to its highest setting. Lay the fillets, skin side up, on the baking sheet. Grill for about 5 minutes, until the skin is crispy and slightly blackened in parts. A skewer should go through it all with no resistance.

While the trout is cooking, put the peas into a microwaveable bowl with a few tablespoons of water. Cover with clingfilm and cook on high for four minutes. Drain well and stir in the pesto.

Take the warmed plates out of the oven, lay the trout fillets on them and you should find that the skin lifts off all in one piece (use a serving platter if you have cooked a whole trout). Place a few slices of lemon on top of the fish, spoon the peas on the side, and sprinkle the fresh basil over it all.

Per serving:

Carbs	23.8g
Proteins	28.7g
Fat	6.25g
Calories	283

Baked Fish with Steamed Leeks in a Crème Fraîche and Chive Sauce

Serves 2

This is another deliciously simple dish. Don't be tempted to use more than the specified amount of crème fraîche, or you'll lose the natural sweetness of the leeks.

Prep time: 5 minutes
Cooking time: 15 minutes

2 good thick fillets of white fish, from the head end
(haddock, hake, coley): 125g per portion
1 lemon, sliced
4 bay leaves
2 large leeks (100g), trimmed, washed and sliced
2 tbsp (20g) half-fat crème fraîche
10 chives, snipped
½ tsp salt
Several good grindings of black pepper

Preheat the oven to 200°C/400°F/Gas Mark 6. Place the fish fillets, skin side down, on a piece of baking parchment and place this on a large sheet of tinfoil.

Put 2 slices of lemon on each fillet along with 2 bay leaves. Wrap the tinfoil loosely over the fish so that it doesn't touch it, but make sure it's as airtight as possible so that the fish steams in the lovely lemony-bay juices. Place in the top of the oven for 15 minutes.

Five minutes before serving, heat a non-stick frying pan and add the leeks. The water from washing them will begin to steam them, so you don't need any oil. Stir-fry them over a medium-high heat until they have softened to the consistency you like. Stir in the crème fraîche, half the chives, and the salt and pepper.

Pile the leeks on the plate and top with a fillet of fish. Pour any remaining baking juices from the fish over it all, and sprinkle the rest of the chives over the top.

Per serving:

Carbs	1.9g
Proteins	24.85g
Fat	2.6g
Calories	137

Golden Fish Chowder

Serves 2

Try to find undyed smoked haddock for this dish (it has a slightly milder taste that works better here) but don't be put off if you can't.

Prep time: 5 minutes
Cooking time: 20 minutes

100g undyed smoked haddock
150g fresh or frozen haddock (thoroughly defrosted if
    frozen)
200ml semi-skimmed milk
300ml water
300g frozen or canned sweetcorn
1 tsp fennel seeds
3 bay leaves
1 tsp fish sauce or ½ tsp anchovy essence
1–2 limes, depending on juiciness
1 spring onion or a few chives, finely chopped

Put both types of haddock in a large pan with the milk and water. Bring to the boil and simmer for 5 minutes. Remove the fish with a sieve and put to one side to cool a little. Add the canned or frozen sweetcorn, fennel seeds, bay leaves and fish sauce to the infused milk, bring to the boil again and simmer for 15 minutes. While this is simmering, remove any skin and bones from the fish and flake it roughly.

After 15 minutes, remove the bay leaves and blend the soup with a freestanding or handheld blender. When it has reached the consistency you like (some people prefer it to be smooth, some prefer there to be whole kernels of corn in it), add the flaked fish and reheat gently. Stir in the juice of 1 lime before checking the taste. Add more lime juice before you add more salt: it's a zingy sort of soup.

Serve in large bowls, garnished with the chopped spring onion or chives.

Per serving:

Carbs	28.0g
Proteins	37.8g
Fat	4.1g
Calories	290

Grilled Mackerel with Apple Sauce and Spinach Salad

Serves 2

Fresh mackerel is perfectly complemented by the tart apple sauce and orangey salad dressing. One of the cheapest fish around, mackerel is full of healthy omega-3 fatty acids.

Prep time: 10 minutes
Cooking time: 20 minutes

1 large cooking apple (200g)
3 tbsp olive oil
2 juicy oranges (200g in total)
2 large or 4 small mackerel (125g per portion), cleaned
5 sprigs rosemary
¼ tsp salt
1 tbsp balsamic vinegar
1 bag washed baby spinach
25g pumpkin seeds or walnuts

First, make the apple sauce. Peel and core the cooking apple, and put it in a heavy-bottomed saucepan with 1 tbsp olive oil and the juice of half an orange. Heat very gently with the lid on for about 10 minutes, stirring from time to time to make sure it doesn't stick and burn. When it's ready, turn the heat right down until you're ready to serve.

Heat the grill to high, and cover the grill pan with a layer of tinfoil to make washing up easier. Place a sprig of rosemary inside each fish and lay them on the tinfoil. If the mackerel are large, make a couple of diagonal slashes on each side so that they cook evenly. Pop them under the grill for 4–5 minutes on each side.

While the mackerel are cooking, mix the rest of the olive oil with the salt, balsamic vinegar and juice of the remaining half orange, and pour into a salad bowl. Peel the second orange and cut into small chunks, removing pips as you go. Toss the chopped orange in the dressing with the spinach leaves and pumpkin seeds or walnuts.

Serve the mackerel with a spoonful of apple sauce on the side, and follow with the spinach salad.

Per serving:

Carbs	12.65g
Proteins	26.3g
Fat	37.95g
Calories	408

Scrambled Eggs with Smoked Salmon and a Cucumber and Dill Salad

Serves 2

This is a classic brunch combination, but I enjoy it just as much at supper time with a crisp salad. Smoked salmon freezes well and defrosts quickly, so if you buy more than you need at one sitting, wrap some of it in clingfilm and put it in the freezer. The dill gives a Swedish flavour to the meal: if you haven't tried it before, just use half a teaspoon as it has quite a strong taste.

Remember that smoked salmon contains salt, so leave it out of the scrambled eggs and you will find you enjoy the contrast of the creamy eggs with the salty salmon.

Prep time: 5 minutes
Cooking time: 5 minutes

6 slices smoked salmon (150g in total)

4 medium eggs

4 tbsp semi-skimmed milk

A few grindings of black pepper

For the cucumber salad:

½ a cucumber (300g), washed and sliced or cut into chunks

1 tsp chopped fresh dill or ½ tsp dried dill

½ tsp olive oil

½ tsp white wine vinegar

Make the salad first: mix all the ingredients together and set aside for a few minutes. Lay the smoked salmon slices on the plates in readiness.

In a heavy-bottomed pan, whisk together the eggs, milk, salt and pepper. Scrambled eggs are best if cooked slowly, so put them over a gentle heat and stir frequently. As soon as the eggs are ready, tip them out onto the plates and give both them and the salmon a few grindings of black pepper.

Serve the cucumber and dill salad on the side, or eat it afterwards.

Per serving:

Carbs	3.5g
Proteins	35.5g
Fat	16.5g
Calories	318

Seafood Stew with Tomato, Fennel and Orange

Serves 2

You can vary the types of seafood you use in this, or you could use one type of fish alone. Tomato, fennel and orange may seem like a strange combination, but believe me it works really well!

Prep time   5 minutes
Cooking time: 20 minutes

1 medium onion (100g)
1 medium carrot (50g)
1 bulb fennel (100g)
1 celery stick
2 tbsp olive oil
1 tsp fennel seeds
125ml orange juice
1 x 410g can chopped tomatoes in their own juice
250ml fresh fish stock (most supermarkets now stock this,
    generally in the chill cabinet near the fish section)
200g bag frozen mixed seafood, defrosted thoroughly;
    or 200g white fish (haddock, monkfish, cod), cut
    into bite-sized chunks

Put the canned tomatoes in a sieve to get rid of some of the excess juice. Peel the onion and carrot and remove any bruised and brown bits from the fennel bulb. Cut off the fennel fronds and set aside for a garnish. Slice the fennel bulb in half and remove the hard core. Trim the celery. With the slicing disc of the food processor, chop the vegetables finely – or do it by hand.

Heat the olive oil in a heavy-bottomed pan and gently fry the vegetables and fennel seeds for a few minutes until the onion turns translucent. Add the orange juice, tinned tomatoes and fish stock. Bring to the boil and simmer gently for 15 minutes. Taste and see if you need to add any more orange juice, or any salt.

Just before serving, tip the seafood into the soup base and stir well. Bring it back to the boil and simmer for 5 minutes to make sure the seafood is thoroughly cooked. Serve in big bowls, garnished with the chopped fennel fronds.

Per serving:

Carbs	19.8g
Proteins	23.75g
Fat	6.3g
Calories	216

VEGETARIAN DISHES

Curried Mushrooms with Gingery Dhal and Creamy Spinach

Serves 2

This is a really warming and filling dish, but dead easy to do. There are some delicious curry pastes on the market now: for this dish you should use tikka masala, vindaloo or moglai rather than anything with coconut or almond. I used the Gujerati Moglai paste by Veeraswamy, which is delicious, but feel free to experiment with your favourite flavours. You can use all button mushrooms, but it's nice to use half button and half chestnut mushrooms. Don't use exotic mushrooms or the large flat Portobello varieties, as they fall apart when you cook them.

Prep time: 5 minutes
Cooking time: 25 minutes

For the mushroom curry:
2 tsp groundnut oil (this gives a nicer flavour – but
    olive oil will do)
1 medium onion (200g), halved and thinly sliced
400g mushrooms, sliced
1 x 410g can chopped tomatoes in their own juice
4 tbsp (28g) curry paste
A few chopped fresh coriander leaves (to garnish)

For the dhal:

1 tsp groundnut oil

1 tsp (6g) garlic purée

1 heaped tbsp (15g) ginger purée

250g red lentils

1 tsp salt

Handful of fresh coriander leaves, finely chopped

For the spinach:

250g frozen spinach

1 tsp groundnut oil

2 tbsp low-fat plain yoghurt

1 tsp curry paste (the same as used for the
   mushrooms)

First, start the mushroom curry. Heat the oil in a heavy-based saucepan and fry the onion over quite a high heat until it begins to brown. Add the mushrooms, tinned tomatoes and curry paste, and stir well. Turn the heat down to a gentle simmer and cook, with the lid off, while you finish the rest of the meal.

For the dhal, you will need a pan with a close-fitting lid. Heat the groundnut oil over a medium heat, then stir in the garlic and ginger purées. Fry for a minute or so, then add the lentils and stir well. Pour in 500ml of cold water, bring to the boil and simmer gently for 20 minutes. You will need to check the dhal after 15 minutes to see if you need to add water. When it has turned to a nice thick consistency, add the salt and coriander leaves and stir well.

Put the spinach into a microwaveable bowl, add a splash of water, cover with clingfilm and microwave on high for 3½ minutes. Uncover, drain well, then stir in the oil, yoghurt and curry paste. You may need to return it to the microwave to reheat: don't overcook or the yoghurt will separate. Serve all three dishes together, sprinkling the fresh coriander leaves over the mushrooms.

Per serving:

Carbs	53.0g
Proteins	20.7g
Fat	6.75g
Calories	273

Roast Butternut Squash with Smoked Tofu and a Red Pepper Sauce

Serves 2

Although this recipe takes 40 minutes, it's well worth waiting for, and the smoked tofu gives it all a lovely barbecue flavour. It also looks absolutely stunning with all the vibrant colours. If you can't find smoked tofu, use plain firm tofu instead and add a pinch of smoked paprika. If you store tofu in the freezer it makes it firmer and less likely to fall apart when you cook it.

Prep time: 10 minutes
Cooking time: 30 minutes

½ a medium butternut squash (400g)
2 tbsp olive oil
1 pot (250ml) roasted red pepper pasta sauce
110g smoked tofu, cut into thin slices or small cubes
100g green beans
15g flaked almonds (to serve)

Preheat the oven to 200°C/400°F/Gas Mark 6.

The skin of butternut squash is perfectly edible, so scrub it well before cutting off the top and bottom ends with a sharp knife. Slice it in half lengthways, and remove the seeds with a spoon. Cut the flesh into ½-inch dice, toss with 1 tbsp olive oil and put on a baking tray. Put the tray in the top of the oven and roast for 20 minutes. Put the pasta sauce and smoked tofu into a small saucepan and simmer very gently so that the tofu doesn't break up as it cooks.

After the squash has roasted for 20 minutes, remove it from the oven and carefully flip the slices with a spatula. Return to the oven for another 10 minutes until the edges begin to caramelize.

Top and tail the beans, and put in a microwaveable bowl with a few tablespoons of water. Cover with clingfilm, microwave on high for 3 minutes, then drain.

Arrange the beans in a layer on the plates, and lay the roasted butternut squash on top. Pour the tofu-rich sauce over, and sprinkle with the flaked almonds.

Per serving:

Carbs	27g
Proteins	20g
Fat	16g
Calories	269

Griddled Aubergine with a Green Salad and Lemon Feta Dressing

Serves 2

This is delicious, and the lemon feta dressing goes well with all sorts of salads. Try it drizzled over ripe tomatoes with a few chives snipped over the top, and put this in pitta bread for lunch the next day. Quark is a very low-fat cheese which is also delicious dolloped over stewed or fresh fruit as a substitute for fromage frais or cream.

Prep time: 5 minutes
Cooking time: 5 minutes

For the dressing:
100g feta cheese
100g Quark
Juice of 1 lemon
Several grindings of black pepper

1 bag rocket, watercress and spinach salad (100g)
30g pine nuts
1 large or 2 medium aubergines (200g)
1 tbsp olive oil
1 tsp thyme leaves

First, make the dressing. Whiz the feta, Quark, lemon juice and black pepper in a food processor, adding just enough water to make it into a creamy sauce. Set aside. Wash the salad, dry it and sprinkle the pine nuts over the leaves.

Heat a ridged frying pan, or turn the grill onto high. Top and tail the aubergines and cut them into ½-inch slices along their length. With a pastry brush, paint them thinly with the olive oil: they will absorb huge amounts if you let them, so go carefully.

Fry or grill the aubergines until they are slightly blackened on each side (about 4–5 minutes). Remove to a plate and sprinkle with the thyme leaves. Pile the salad on the side and drizzle the creamy dressing over everything.

Per serving:

Carbs	5.8g
Proteins	18.5g
Fat	23.4g
Calories	311

Speckled Salad with Lemon Feta Dressing

Serves 2

Use the dressing from the recipe for griddled aubergine, page 244, as a basis for this prettiest of summer salads, full of crunch and goodness. Vary the ingredients to suit your taste, but I think this is a nice combination.

1 medium carrot (150g)

3 radishes

2 sticks celery

¼ cucumber (150g)

2 tbsp (20g) pumpkin seeds

1 tbsp (10g) pine nuts

25g feta cheese (a ½-inch slice)

3 tbsp lemon feta dressing (see recipe for griddled
    aubergine, page 244)

1 dessert apple (150g): Braeburn, Jazz, Pink Lady or
    Cox's are all good

Salt and pepper to taste

1 bag rocket leaves (100g), washed and well spun

Peel the carrot and chop into small chunks. Top and tail the radishes and celery and chop into similar-sized chunks. Scrub the skin of the cucumber and, with a teaspoon, scrape out the seeds – this stops the salad getting too watery. In a small saucepan over a medium heat, dry-fry the pumpkin seeds and pine nuts until beginning to brown (you can skip this step if you're in a hurry). Mix all the vegetables with the nuts and seeds in a bowl and crumble in the feta cheese. Add 2 tbsp lemon feta dressing and mix well. Core the apple and cut into chunks, slices or whatever takes your fancy, before adding it to the salad. Mix well: you add the apple last to stop it browning on contact with the air. Taste the salad: you may want to add more lemon juice, a little salt or a few grinds of pepper.

Put the salad leaves onto plates, and place a mound of salad in the middle. Drizzle the rest of the dressing over the green leaves.

Per serving:

Carbs	13.15g
Proteins	6.2g
Fat	8.15g
Calories	168

Chickpea Soup with Sun-dried Tomatoes

Serves 4

This is a very easy, tasty, satisfying soup which freezes beautifully. Non-vegetarians can substitute a slice of crispy bacon, grilled and crumbled, for the sun-dried tomatoes. If you can find them, use semi-dried tomatoes from the deli counter: they're full of herby flavours.

Prep time: 5 minutes
Cooking time: 10 minutes

3 x 410g cans chickpeas
2 sprigs rosemary
2 white onions (150g), peeled and finely chopped
4 cloves garlic, peeled and finely chopped
1 x 410g can chopped tomatoes in their own juice
4 sun-dried tomatoes
1 tsp Marigold vegetable bouillon powder, or ½ a
    vegetable stock cube
Salt and pepper to taste
20g grated Parmesan
15g flat-leaf parsley, finely chopped
Few drops of chilli oil
2 tsp extra virgin olive oil

Rinse the chickpeas under cold water. Add them to a large soup pot with the rosemary, chopped onions, chopped garlic, tinned tomatoes, sun-dried tomatoes, bouillon powder or stock cube, and enough cold water to cover generously. Bring to the boil and simmer gently for 10 minutes.

The soup will be ready for the next step when the onion is soft. Remove half the soup to a blender and whiz till smooth before returning it to the pan and stirring in, or use a hand-held blender to get it to the consistency you like. Bring the soup back to a simmer: taste and season, but don't add too much salt as you'll get this from the Parmesan.

At the last moment, dish the soup into the bowls. Sprinkle a little Parmesan and parsley into each bowl; dot the chilli oil and half a teaspoon of extra virgin olive oil around each bowl to give a lovely flavour.

Per serving:

Carbs	55.0g
Proteins	23.0g
Fat	14.7g
Calories	355

Super-simple Vegetarian Chilli with Lime and Coriander

Serves 2

There are many good chilli sauces on the market, but it's fun to tart them up with your own ingredients. You'll be amazed how fresh the chilli tastes if you make up your own spice mix, and Quorn is a good base for soaking up the highly flavoured sauce. Remember to check how hot the chilli sauce is before adding any more Tabasco!

Prep time: 5 minutes to 2 hours, depending
on how much time you have
Cooking time: 20 minutes

1 tbsp dried oregano

2 tsp sweet paprika

1 tsp cumin seeds

1 tbsp coriander seeds

250g Quorn chunks

350g chilli sauce (I used the Discovery range, which is
very nice indeed)

3 sun-dried tomatoes, chopped

1 medium red onion (200g), peeled and chopped

2 cloves garlic, peeled and chopped

1 can mixed bean salad
Salt and pepper to taste
Juice of 1 lime

To serve:
125ml low-fat plain yoghurt
30g fresh coriander, washed and chopped
Tabasco sauce

In a coffee grinder or mortar and pestle, grind together the coriander seeds, oregano, paprika and cumin. Sprinkle the spice mix over the Quorn chunks, mix well and set aside for anything up to 2 hours.

In a heavy-bottomed saucepan, mix together the chilli sauce, sun-dried tomatoes, onion and garlic. Bring to the boil and simmer for 10 minutes. Add the beans and Quorn and simmer for a further 15 minutes with the lid off, stirring fairly frequently to stop it sticking. Season and stir in the lime juice right at the end.

Serve in big bowls with a tablespoon of low-fat yoghurt in the middle and a sprinkling of chopped fresh coriander. A few drops of Tabasco look pretty, but don't overdo it!

Per serving:

Carbs	55.0g
Proteins	26.8g
Fat	14.1g
Calories	343

Full of Goodness (FOG) Soup

Makes 1 week's worth

This recipe first appeared in my book *Drop a Size in 2 Weeks Flat!* I received so many e-mails from readers telling me how much they liked it that I've included it again here. It really is delicious and filling.

Choose at least five of the vegetables listed below – the more the merrier! The initial preparation and cooking takes a little while, but you then have a convenient soup that will last a week in the fridge – it freezes well too.

1 onion, coarsely chopped

1 courgette, coarsely chopped

Handful of green beans, cut into 1.5-cm lengths

1 carrot, diced

3 sticks celery, peeled with a potato peeler to remove the ridged strands, then coarsely chopped

1 leek, coarsely chopped

¼ cauliflower, cut into small, bite-sized pieces

4–5 green cabbage or spring green leaves, sliced into strips

1 small bunch broccoli, cut into small, bite-sized pieces

1 parsnip, peeled and cut into bite-sized pieces

400g can cannellini beans, drained and rinsed

Handful of frozen peas

Handful of mangetout, diced

4–5 dried mushrooms, softened in 280ml boiling water
   (the water can be added to the soup)

4 chicken or vegetable stock cubes

Good handful of fresh chopped flat-leaf or curly parsley

Put all the vegetables, beans and peas into a big stock pan, together with the stock cubes and 4 litres of cold water. Bring to the boil, then simmer on a very low heat, covered, for about 2 hours. Season well, halfway through cooking time.

Whiz half of the soup in a blender or liquidizer and return to the pot. Throw in the chopped parsley and serve.

CLIENT FEEDBACK: LOUISE

Testing these recipes has completely changed the way I eat. I don't have a problem with my weight but I used to have a real craving in the evening for a glass of wine and some crisps or nuts as I was preparing supper. One glass led to two, and before I knew it I was slumped in front of the telly feeling very full, slightly sloshed and cross that I was watching rubbish again.

I would be fine the next day until the evening. I've always had a relatively light lunch, and am quite good at not picking at the kids' supper. But by the time I was ready to eat supper I was starving, hence the crisps and the wine. Not any more! Now I wake up quite hungry and happily eat a large breakfast (toast and marmalade, sometimes with muesli as well) that sees me through to lunch. I haven't changed my lunch, but knowing that I'm not going to eat carbs for supper means I don't worry about having something at teatime such as a couple of biscuits and some fruit or a toasted teacake. This keeps me going until well into the evening because I'm not desperately hungry. I'm sleeping better and have more energy – from a simple change in my diet!

11

Stop a Lapse Becoming a Collapse

So you have slipped off the plan a little ... the first thing is not to panic! You haven't failed, and coming a little unstuck is to be expected. So stop beating yourself up and let's get back on track. Remember, we are building a Template of Success, not a Template of Failure (see Chapter 1), and you are not about to cop out of your plan.

Here's how to stop your lapse becoming a collapse:

1. Double Carb Curfew

For a maximum of two days you can do a double Carb Curfew. So omit your carbs not just after 5pm but also at either your lunch or your breakfast. Not at both.

66 I got a lot of comfort from the fact that if I did have a blowout I could follow the eating principles strictly. 99

2. Do the Step Trade-off

OK, so you arrive at work famished, and the biscuits are just too good to resist – allow yourself to have one, but before you eat it check out what it is going to cost you in additional steps or walking today. The information in Chapter 9 on page 201 will help you work this out.

3. Play the '300 Game'

If you have overindulged then cut your calorie intake by 300 calories the following day and add an extra 10 minutes to your walk. This will create an additional 400 calorie burn, which will help get you back on track. The slight decrease in calories combined with slow-releasing carbohydrates will help keep you in control and stop you feeling ravenous the following day, when you may just want to hoover every morsel of food you see. In addition, your walking will help even out your blood sugar levels, stabilizing your moods and keeping your body burning calories throughout the day.

PLAY THE 300 GAME IN ADVANCE

A party, wedding or other big social event can make it difficult to stick to the plan. If you know a particular day is going to be hard, plan ahead a little. The day before your potential cop-out day eat 300 fewer calories and add 10 minutes' walking to your daily target. Repeat this the day after the event and you'll soon see you are back on track, catching up and not copping out.

---

4. Visit Your Motivation Box

In Chapter 7 I asked you to write down five reasons why you wanted to lose weight and to put them in a box. Now is the time to visit that box!

Pick out one of your reminders – read it and focus on why you wrote that as motivation for your plan. Place it back in the box and, on a fresh piece of paper, write a new motivation for keeping on track.

5. Reaffirm Your Positive Affirmations

Before you twist that knife even further into your back, or run to the fridge to seek solace in food, read through all the ways you can be nice to yourself, below. OK, so you did cop out, but being brutally cruel to yourself and stuffing your face with food is not going to help you catch up. You'll wake up with a food hangover and make it harder for your cells to use calories and nutrients effectively.

LET ME COUNT THE WAYS ... TO BE GOOD TO MYSELF

Soak in the bathtub

Plan my career

Collect shells

Recycle old items

Go on a date

Buy flowers

Go to a movie in the middle of the week

Walk or jog

Listen to music

Recall past parties

Buy household gadgets

Read a humorous book

Think about my past trips

Listen to others

Read magazines or newspapers

Do some woodwork

Build a model

Spend an evening with good friends

Meet new people

Remember beautiful scenery

Save money

Go home from work

Practise karate, judo or yoga

Think about retirement

Repair things

Work on my car or bicycle

Remember the words and deeds of loving people

Wear sexy clothes

Ride a motorcycle

Practise religion (go to church, pray)

Go to the beach

Sing around the house

Go skating

Paint

Do needlepoint, knitting, sewing, etc.

Take a nap

Entertain

Go to a club meeting

Sing with groups

Flirt

Play a musical instrument

Make a gift for someone

Collect postcards

Buy a CD

Plan a party

Go hiking

Write a love poem

Buy clothes

Go sightseeing

Garden

Go to the beauty salon or hairdresser

Buy a book

Watch children play

Write a letter
Write in a diary
Go to a play or concert
Daydream
Go to the mountains
Think about happy moments in my childhood
See or show photographs or slides
Play cards, chess, draughts etc.
Solve riddles
Have a political discussion
Do crossword puzzles
Shoot pool
Dress up and look nice
Think about how I've improved
Buy something for myself (perfume, golf balls, etc.)
Talk on the phone
Kiss
Go to a museum
Light candles
Have a massage
Say 'I love you'
Take a sauna or steam bath
Go skiing
Visit an aquarium
Go horse riding
Do a jigsaw puzzle
Go window shopping
Send a greetings card to someone I care about

6. Commit to Filling in Your Food Diaries

This may seem a burden but committing yourself to writing everything down will keep you on track. Take your food charts and mark off each day.

7. Be an Early Bird

Try to take your walk first thing in the morning. This will help get your head in the right space, and the feel-good factor will have a positive knock-on effect on your eating and activity right through the day. Studies have clearly shown that people who take their exercise first thing in the morning are still following their exercise programme 12 months later.

DON'T DO THE STUFF AND STARVE

If you had a blowout yesterday, don't do the stuff and starve! Starving yourself today in an effort to 'catch up on your extra calories' is false economy for two reasons:

1 Your overindulgence from the day before will most likely have thrown your blood sugar levels into disarray, which will make you feel more hungry, more irritable or even more erratic.
2 Starving yourself and depriving yourself of food today will only serve to throw your blood sugars out further and take them longer to stabilize. Instead, play the 300 game (see page 257).

If you have to eat business lunches out you don't need to feel really guilty as you know you can either swap the Carb Curfew meals or eat fewer carbs the next day.

12

Questions and Answers

As you go through the 28-day programme you may well have some questions. Below you'll find some commonly asked questions and their answers. You will also find some tips in the questions-and-answers section of my website: www.joannahall.com

I know I should eat breakfast but if I do it makes me feel hungry all day and I can't stop eating.

This may be because you are not getting enough protein in your breakfast. Protein helps stimulate the release of dopamine in the brain, making you feel more alert. So it is important to have a serving of protein with your breakfast. Your hunger cravings may also be misguided: your body may actually require water, not sugar, so your breakfast is also an important opportunity to hydrate your body.

Consuming some wholegrain, rather than refined, carbohydrate for breakfast will fuel your brain and your nervous system, help preserve your lean muscle tissue and provide fibre and nutrients.

Eating the right carbohydrate is important to maximize your energy and your weight loss. Your breakfast choices need to be built around low- to moderate-Glycaemic Index carbohydrates (see table on page 55). You will probably notice that bread, which is considered a staple of our diet, is a high-GI carb, but don't panic. If you really are a bread lover, eating some protein and a little fat with it will slow down the release of blood sugar and create more of a low- to moderate-GI response.

I have heard that I should be active for 30 minutes a day, for five or more days a week. How does this fit in with the 10,000 steps message?

This is still valid. Walking briskly for 30 minutes a day has been proven to reduce the risk of disease in many areas. It is the current guideline given by most UK and US health organizations. It has also been shown that the 30 minutes can be split into two lots of 15 minutes, or three lots of 10 minutes, and still bring significant health benefits.

Getting started with a physical activity routine is a major step on the way to an active lifestyle. Unfortunately, we cannot bottle the benefits from our current exercise habits for use at some point in the future. Physical activity has to be sustained over the longer term to accrue the significant health benefits associated with it. Even former athletes who quit exercise altogether at the end of their careers have similar rates of chronic disease as people who've never exercised. Finding a physical activity routine that you can sustain throughout your life is critical for deriving maximum benefit. Importantly, it's never too late to start. People who take up exercise in their 60s can still achieve significant health benefits.

Will I lose weight just by doing the walking programme?

The daily walking target of 10,000 steps is widely recognized as the target to aim for to see improvements in your health and weight management. But while taking 10,000 steps a day can improve your fitness, without any dietary changes it will not be enough for you to see weight loss. So if your primary aim is to lose weight, you will need to follow the Carb Curfew plan as well as the walking targets. However, if you feel you may find it difficult to cope with both the walking and the diet, then just follow the walking plan. You will definitely feel better, see improvements in your body shape, and your clothes should fit you better. Some of my clients have completed the 28-day programme just focusing on the walking. The improvements they experience in their confidence, self-esteem, and energy levels – and comments from friends about how much better they look – have given them the confidence to start another 28-day plan, this time addressing the diet as well.

Taking 10,000–12,000 steps a day and changing your eating habits will result in weight loss and inch loss. If you want to experience weight loss but are not prepared to adjust your eating habits, studies have shown you will need to take in the region of 20,000 steps a day. Even without weight loss, regular moderate exercise will reduce your abdominal fat and insulin resistance. This improved fitness is important for decreasing your risk of chronic diseases. So even if you do not decrease your total weight by following my 28-day walking programme, you will alter your abdominal fat and get great health outcomes.

Does a high-protein diet work for long-term weight loss?

A study analysing two groups over 12 months found the group who followed a moderate carbohydrate and lower protein intake kept the weight off compared to the group who followed a high-protein, low-carbohydrate diet. Bottom line – don't cut out all your carbs!

I seem to just glance at a bowl of pasta and I've gained 4 pounds, and when I stand on the scales – there they are looking straight up at me!

This is something I often come across with clients before they start the Carb Curfew plan. Your body has not miraculously gained 4 pounds of body fat overnight. For your body to gain this amount of weight you would have had to eat an additional 14,000 calories a day on top of your normal intake. That's equivalent to 46 double chocolate chip muffins! But you may have gained a pound, and if those additional calories have come from starchy carbs they will naturally hold on to three units of water.

CLIENT FEEDBACK: JUDY

Portion distortion has changed my life – I have never felt better. It is so clever, simple and easy to do that no one need ever know you are following a diet. I have been on so many diets in the past – as a grandma, that's quite a few years of dieting! I have always found them depressing and, while I have had a bit of success, it's always been a chore. I gave up smoking seven years ago and the weight piled on. Now, after Joanna's 28-day plan, I have lost so many inches, but I look healthy and well and shapely – not drawn. I am a new woman – and that's saying something since I'm in my 60s!

I love my pedometer. The daily walking targets kept me on track and became part of my everyday life in a very short time. My family can't believe how much happier and positive I am – I have so much more energy now to enjoy my grandchildren – all seven of them!

DROP A SIZE IN TWO WEEKS FLAT!

The Quick Fix You're Looking for to Get you into Your Jeans, Your Bikini, or that Little Black Dress

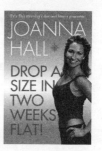

Joanna Hall offers you the quick and healthy way to drop a dress size as well as the solution to long-term weight management so you can look good every day of the year.

- ✪ **Use the Carb Curfew plan**
- ✪ **Which carbs to choose and when to eat them**
- ✪ **Exercise to get your rear in gear**
- ✪ **Fantastic, easy recipes**
- ✪ **How to use 'Habit Grooving' to make the plan a way of life**

CARB CURFEW

Cut the Carbs after 5pm and Lose Fat Fast!

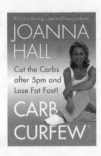

Joanna Hall's *Carb Curfew* is a highly effective and practical diet and fitness plan. It is flexible to fit with your life, however hectic it is, so that you can maintain your weight loss over the long term.

- ✪ **How to follow Joanna's Carb Curfew plan**
- ✪ **Why you should drink 2 litres of water a day**
- ✪ **Why eating the right fats can help your body lose fat**
- ✪ **How to build activity into your day**
- ✪ **Use the 80/20 rule – be consistent 80% of the time**

Using these five steps you can really change your level of fitness. And with the delicious selection of Carb Curfew recipes you'll lose weight fast.

DROP A SIZE FOR LIFE

Fat Loss – Fast and Forever!

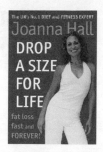

Drop a size and keep it off, whatever life throws at you!

A quick-fix diet is a 'one-night-stand' in nutritional terms. *Drop a Size for Life* will be your compatible partner for life!

Joanna's groundbreaking *Carb Curfew* plan has been described as the most healthy and effective alternative to typical high protein diets, including Dr Atkins'.

- ✪ **Get active and you'll stay in shape for years, not just weeks**
- ✪ **Use Joanna's mental strategies to keep on track**
- ✪ **Eat Joanna's Carb Curfew meals – and never go hungry**

When life has a habit of throwing obstacles in your path such as work stress, parties, holidays, pregnancy or menopause, Joanna Hall offers the strategies you need to resist those rebound pounds for good!

DROP A SIZE CARB AND CALORIE COUNTER

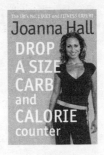

Joanna Hall's carb and calorie counter is the must-have companion to her Carb Curfew programme as well as any other low-carb plan.

It gives you the calorie, carb, fat, protein and fibre content of over 5,000 foods, snacks, drinks and supermarket ready meals. Joanna also explains:

- ✪ **How Carb Curfew works**
- ✪ **Which foods are particularly rich in vitamins and minerals**
- ✪ **Why many food labels are misleading**
- ✪ **Which carbs and fats are healthiest**
- ✪ **Why portion size is a key issue**

Easy to use and jam-packed with information, this book is essential to your achieving a healthy weight and fabulous figure.

Make
www.thorsonselement.com
your online sanctuary

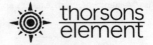